SHORTEST HISTORY

HISTORY

OF

EUGENICS

From "Science" to Atrocity—How a
Dangerous Movement Shaped the
World, and Why It Persists

ERIK L. PETERSON

THE EXPERIMENT

NEW YORK

The Experiment, LLC
220 East 23rd Street, Suite 600
New York, NY 10010-4658
theexperimentpublishing.com

THE EXPERIMENT and its colophon are registered trademarks of The Experiment, LLC. Many of the designations used by manufacturers and sellers to distinguish their products are claimed as trademarks. Where those designations appear in this book and The Experiment was aware of a trademark claim, the designations have been capitalized.

The Experiment's books are available at special discounts when purchased in bulk for premiums and sales promotions as well as for fundraising or educational use. For details, contact us at info@theexperimentpublishing.com.

Library of Congress Cataloging-in-Publication Data

Names: Peterson, Erik L., author.
Title: The shortest history of eugenics : from "science" to atrocity - how a dangerous movement shaped the world, and why it persists / Erik L. Peterson.
Description: New York : The Experiment, [2024] | Series: The shortest history series | Includes bibliographical references and index.
Identifiers: LCCN 2024036600 (print) | LCCN 2024036601 (ebook) | ISBN 9781891011887 (paperback) | ISBN 9781891011870 (ebook)
Subjects: LCSH: Eugenics--History.
Classification: LCC HQ751 .P44 2024 (print) | LCC HQ751 (ebook) | DDC 363.9/2--dc23/eng/20240816
LC record available at https://lccn.loc.gov/2024036600
LC ebook record available at https://lccn.loc.gov/2024036601

ISBN 978-1-891011-88-7
Ebook ISBN 978-1-891011-87-0

Cover design by Jack Dunnington
Text design by Beth Bugler

Manufactured in the United States of America

First printing December 2024
10 9 8 7 6 5 4 3 2 1

To Cathy Caldwell Hoop and John M. McCollum, who have shown me what a more just world looks like

Contents

Preface: The Good Birth

What do we mean by "eugenics"? Perhaps you've picked up this book because you're curious about this strange word in the title. Let me address that right away: It's a Greek word, and it just means "well born" or "good birth." In that sense, it seems innocent enough. After all, we all want more healthy babies to be brought into the world, right?

But I suspect you're here because you've heard that this word has other connotations. Sinister ones. Maybe you have images of mad scientists and Nazi physicians in your mind right now. And you would be right. The story of eugenics is tragic, even horrific. Indeed, Nazi doctors are definitely among the villains in this story.

The reason I'm writing this book, however, is because, though the Third Reich fell, never to return, I'm not convinced that we've turned the last page on the eugenics story. Eugenics, in other words, may be *forgotten*, but it's not *gone*.

Aha!, you might be thinking, *This will be a book about "playing God" with "designer babies."* You might think I will be warning you of shiny new biotech like CRISPR and artificial wombs that will allow people to select particular traits, even enhancements, that they prefer in their offspring—that someday soon we will end up with a group of genetic "haves" and another of genetic "have-nots." If I were writing that sort of a book, I would be in a crowded landscape. This has been a popular worry for decades. One of my favorite films from the 1990s, *Gattaca*, has this concern as its core theme. Now some well-known scientists refer to this as "velvet eugenics," a consumer-driven genetic race for supremacy.

Velvet eugenics grabs our attention. It sounds sci-fi and is the plot of many dystopian movies and books. But sadly, it ignores the actual history of eugenics. This ignorance allows all these worries about velvet eugenics to distract us from the real issues staring us in the face.

Let me start by laying out the traditional history of eugenics. In the last two decades of the 1800s, in Queen Victoria's Britain, there was a scientist named Francis Galton. We often mention that Galton was the cousin of Charles Darwin— they shared a famous grandfather. (This detail both makes the story spicier and fits better with our velvet eugenics fears about evolutionary biology run amok.) Galton thought that some people are born "fit" and others "unfit." The fit should be encouraged to have more babies and the unfit fewer. This is what he called "eugenics" in 1883. Then American scientists and doctors ran with Galton's ideas and practiced them on patients in mental hospitals, sterilizing many thousands. There was even a Supreme Court case about it, *Buck v. Bell* (1927). Right around then, Germany started practicing it too. Soon, Nazis applied these Galtonian ideas about eliminating the unfit to millions during the Holocaust. After the Doctors' Trial at Nuremberg after World War II, scientists realized the error of their ways, disavowing eugenics and experimentation on human subjects. We now have policies in place to ensure that we never do this again in the name of science. Some scholars go a step further, insisting we can only call eugenics a "pseudoscience," weird beliefs costumed up in a lab coat, just to emphasize how well we've learned our lesson about the wrongness of eugenics and how our modern science is on the straight and narrow path toward objectivity.

Most of the above traditional history is true. But it is very, very incomplete. It's those parts forgotten in the dark corners of this canned history that make me fear not sci-fi velvet eugenics but the reemergence and expansion of the real deal. Doing again what we've *already done*. No "pseudo" about it.

So, let's start over. What do we mean by "eugenics"?

Historically, eugenics was actually two things: scientific ideas, on the one hand, and medical techniques and the justifications for their use, on the other. Each had its own separate trajectory, its own history. Each flourished in different places and at different times, often overlapping, but not everywhere all the time.

As we will see in the first chapter, scientific ideas that some are *inherently* healthy, robust, smart, charismatic (the "fit")— and others sickly, weak, mentally impaired, lazy, alcoholics (the "unfit")—and that only the fit should be permitted to breed for the benefit of future generations, is a very old idea. True, Francis Galton repackaged these ideas in the Victorian era, but he didn't invent them. More important, Galton was only one voice among many in that era trying to promote these ideas and apply them to the realities of industrialism, migration, and rapid urbanization. Scientific ideas about unfitness and societal decay swirled in Continental Europe before Galton wrote about them in England. And in the 1870s, an American religious group, the Oneida Bible Commune, successfully built their multigenerational society around these ancient ideas about breeding humans scientifically.

It's the second aspect of eugenics, the adoption of medical techniques and the justifications for their use, where we can begin to see a dark and often unspoken twist in the history. Inhibiting reproduction by altering or destroying the sexual organs was the most notorious medical technique employed by eugenicists in the first half of the twentieth century, though permanent custodial care with little or no possibility of release was the most frequent. Yet the history of this practice remains largely in the background of eugenics histories. Already by the 1850s, before any European scientific concept of "fitness," American physicians recommended "asexualizing" (usually a euphemism for male castration) or "blistering" the thighs or genitals of sexual deviants and criminals, which often included homosexuals and excessive masturbators.[1] It's the explicit justification for these surgeries that was the driver for the darkest parts of eugenics. As one prominent Chicago physician bluntly put it in the *New York Medical Journal*: "Sex Mutilations" could be "a Remedy for Social Ills."

European scientists developed their eugenics ideas alongside a new understanding of genetics. American physicians, on the other hand, pursued what I call "vigilante medicine." Here's what I mean. Physicians enjoyed almost complete autonomy in Gilded Age America following the Civil War. With very little medical training, and even less oversight, they were free to treat the ills of their entire community in whatever ways they saw fit. Violence in pursuit of "justice"—from lynchings to the punishments doled out by self-appointed regulator militias—was common enough in nineteenth-century America. Though we may never know their numbers with certainty, American medical journal publications attest that many physicians took it upon themselves to right society's wrongs with their own surgical knives. As they noted, it was certainly a less violent form of justice than that regularly meted out elsewhere by men with ropes and guns.

It's this bifurcated story about European science on the one hand and American medicine on the other that makes the true history of eugenics so much more extensive, much more an embedded part of American society than how we usually portray it. In the last decade of the nineteenth century, waves of European ideas about heredity and evolutionary fitness crashed onto an American shore that was *already primed* to prescribe surgical solutions for social problems.

And there were *so many* social problems in turn-of-the-century America; in that ecosystem, eugenics flourished. The US became a European-style ocean-spanning colonial empire after encircling or annihilating First Nations in the American West, then acquiring the Hawaiian Islands, the Philippines, Guam, Puerto Rico, and parts of the Caribbean. With the newly acquired ability to harness electromagnetism, factories surged, electric lighting crammed more day into the night, telegraphs and newspapers spawned a transcontinental information glut, and urban areas burst at the seams. European and Asian immigrants and African Americans risked ocean and continent crossing for the hope of American industrial wealth. They also kept wages low and fueled labor actions for better working conditions, some of which turned bloody. Together, these factors amped up fears among the elite and middle-class Anglo-Americans that the burden of caring for the marginalized would fall upon them. Permeating it all: the perennial American mistrust of the non-white Other— whether Chinese, Japanese, Black, Mexican, Native American, Puerto Rican, Filipino, and so on.

Armed with the European scientific notion that society itself might be biologically deteriorating and that these negative biological traits could be carried on invisible genes, American eugenicists argued that the most convenient way to deal with persistent social problems was to eliminate the lineages of those who suffer from them. Cut off the genes. Of course, those with social, economic, political, scientific, and medical power got to decide *who* were the sources of society's suffering. In other words, eugenics has always been about the powerful, wealthy, and connected influencing, if not outright controlling, the reproduction of the less-powerful, poorer, and more marginalized, with scalpels if necessary—*that's* what we mean by eugenics.

Between the two World Wars, American eugenicists spun an enormous web of professional, social, legal, political, and economic connections across the entire planet, funded by some of America's best-known and wealthiest families, corporations, and philanthropic organizations. The scientific ideas and medical techniques of American eugenics traveled quickly along those networks. German scientists paid close attention. By the 1930s, they had adopted many features of American eugenics on their way to the cold mania orchestrating the Holocaust.

Many of the scientific ideas underlying eugenics were discredited in the wake of World War II. Too often, our histories of eugenics end there. It was a pseudoscience; we learned our lesson—end of story.

But pause to examine the medical techniques and their justifications rather than merely the scientific ideas, and you'll see that a surprising amount survived the war, most notably in the US and its new overseas colonies. Through the twentieth century, even after the Nazi atrocities, American physicians and, increasingly, political figures continued to reason that the most convenient way to deal with persistent social problems was to medically inhibit the reproduction of the unwanted. Perhaps unsurprisingly, as the US became one of the world's main political, economic, scientific, and military powers during the Cold War, that conviction about inhibiting reproduction of the unwanted spread across the globe once again. The simultaneous advent of reliable pharmaceutical contraception only made the medical techniques more effective, more efficient, and cheaper. Moreover, pills, intrauterine devices, and injections offered by friendly health care providers just seemed less objectionable than surgeons wielding scalpels in asylums, even if the motivations behind both were largely the same. Controlling the reproduction of the unwanted continued on a global scale, but fewer noticed. Even the ones who did rarely used that fusty old word "eugenics" anymore.

A final note: Eugenics is often mentioned in the same breath with "social Darwinism" and "scientific racism." Additionally, some regard the Tuskegee syphilis trials (1932–1972) as an example of eugenics, despite the fact that no physician suggested curtailing anyone's reproduction. I want to emphasize important distinctions in terms that will become clearer throughout the book.

Eugenics in the twentieth century represented a different kind of racism from what preceded it. Eighteenth- and nineteenth-century scientific racism based on skull comparisons was predicated on explaining—often by reference to biological features of the white body and brain—the military, cultural, intellectual, and political project of European colonialism. Likewise, the "social" Darwinian ideas about dog-eat-dog competition espoused by scientists, politicians, and business-men in the late 1800s justified white supremacy, among other things. European and American militaries and colonists and corporations dominated markets and territory, so went the rhetoric, due to inborn racial superiority. Even the Tuskegee syphilis trials, in which medical professionals refused to offer the most up-to-date treatments to impoverished African American men suffering from syphilis in rural Alabama, were implicitly motivated by feelings that Black lives didn't matter.

By the late nineteenth century, the emphasis of this racism shifted. Rather than emphasizing colonial dominance and commercial prowess, European and American scientists and physicians decried that whites were in demographic danger. Non-whites had more babies. And the fruits of modern medicine and industrialization allowed whites to coddle physically and mentally weak children who would pass those inferior traits on to *their* white babies. In only a few generations, the tax dollars and charitable giving of wealthy whites would be dwarfed by teeming hordes of the ill, criminal, and impoverished. In other words, the racism motivating eugenics was the kind founded on the fear that whites would be sapped of financial resources and then demographically "replaced" by prolific non-whites. And if that term "white replacement" sounds eerily familiar, that's because it has reappeared in online screeds, shouted at tiki-torch race rallies, and even been teased in political speeches.

That's my larger point in this book. The scientific ideas, the medical techniques, and the ideological scaffolding for eugenics did not merely appear a century ago and then disappear in the rubble of World War II. Both the Victorian fears and the early twentieth-century medical "fix" for persistent social problems continue to percolate to the surface even in the twenty-first century. The temptation to fix those problems by controlling the reproduction of the poor and non-white lurks nearby still. The question remains: What will people of good will choose to do with their knowledge of this more complete, if brief, history?

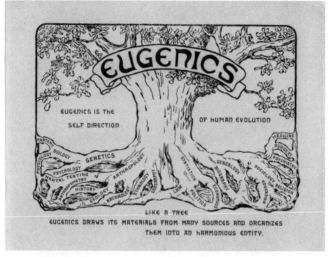

By the twentieth century, advocates symbolized eugenics as an all-encompassing pursuit for human improvement.

PART 1

Surviving the Unfittest

(C. 500 BCE TO 1898)

PART I

Surviving the Darkness
But to 1985

CHAPTER 1

Managing Fate

It often goes unspoken, but the first and most important element of eugenics is the idea that a person is determined or fated toward a certain outcome because of what kind of creature they are, what they carry around inside them—their very essence, their truest self. You can find this very old idea in the Book of Genesis. Ten times the text repeats that God created plants and animals "according to its [or their] kind." Those "kinds" performed certain tasks or produced specific fruit, even, infamously, a fruit that contained "knowledge of good and evil." As the story goes, when our first ancestors consumed that fruit, the knowledge of good and evil passed on to them. All the unforeseen consequences that followed that action became embedded within humanity itself, part of the essence of being human, our shared fate.

Of course, other ancient societies recognized different fates for different kinds of people too. The widely read ancient Greek poet Theognis of Megara, the Richard Dawkins of his day, put it clearly.

We seek out rams and asses and horses that are purebred [. . .] but a noble man does not mind marrying the base daughter of a base father if the latter gives him a lot of money, and a woman does not refuse to be the wife of a base man who is rich [. . .]. It is money people

*honour [. . .] Wealth has mixed up blood. And so,
Polypaïdes, do not be surprised that the townsmen's stock
is becoming enfeebled, since what is* noble *is mixing with
what is base.*[1]

People noble in their very essence were having children
with other people whom Theognis and his peers considered
ignoble. *Blood* now mixed. The result, warned Theognis,
would be *societal* weakness. To avoid this, he preached, we
should apply the same logic to the breeding of human kinds as
we do to the breeding of different kinds of livestock.

Theognis wrote these words around 2,500 years ago—
24 centuries before anyone studied "genetics," let alone "eugenics." But all the ingredients that went into shaping twentieth-
century eugenics are right there in his poetic lament.

- The comparison with livestock breeding
- The worry about essential weakness passing from parent
  to child
- Scolding about mixing up blood, at *sullying the race*
- A call for thoughtful selection of breeding humans in
  order to prevent *biological* corruption

Well, *nearly* all the ingredients. It's true that no less a figure
than Charles Darwin believed that Theognis "clearly saw
how important selection, if carefully applied, would be for
the improvement of mankind"—the sentiment that Darwin's
cousin Francis Galton famously dubbed "eugenics."[2] Yet, other
scholars of ancient Greek poetry disagree with Darwin. They
believe other lines of the long poem reveal that Theognis did
not think blood/biology *determined* the fate of individuals
or whole societies.[3] Perhaps philosopher Frederick Nietzsche,
who studied Theognis as a student, captured the ancient

poet's motivations best. Theognis was mostly just bitter about the lower classes.

"Theognis appears as a finely formed nobleman who has fallen on bad times . . . full of fatal hatred toward the upward striving masses. . . . What is past seems so beautiful and enviable, that which is coming . . . seems disgusting and repulsive; a typical [reaction] for all those noble figures who represent the aristocracy prior to a popular revolution."
—Friedrich Nietzsche, *De Theognide Megarensi* (1864)[4]

Plato, on the other hand, believed in a harder kind of determinism. A century after Theognis, Plato, arguably the most influential philosopher of all time, stipulated in his *Republic* that the ruling classes must arrange marriages so that the best should leave behind the largest number of children for the betterment of all humankind. Then the community should expend resources to rear the offspring of carefully chosen matches but neglect those of the inferior.[5] Not surprisingly, his endorsement of Theognis in *Republic*, one of history's most influential books, resonated through the ages.

Socrates: "How, then, would the greatest benefit result? Tell me this, Glaucon. I see that you have in your house hunting-dogs and a number of pedigree birds. Have you ever considered something about their unions and procreations?" . . . "Do you then breed from all indiscriminately, or are you careful to breed from the best?"

> Glaucon: "From the best." . . .
>
> Socrates: "It follows from our former admissions . . . that the best men must cohabit with the best women in as many cases as possible and the worst with the worst in the fewest, and that the offspring of the one must be reared and that of the other not, if the flock is to be as perfect as possible."
>
> —Plato, *Republic*, Book 5, 459 (c. 375 BCE)[6]

Nevertheless, controlling human breeding for the betterment of society seems not to have registered as a serious solution for centuries. Supposedly, pockets of Greeks and Romans practiced infanticide to cull the disabled. The Roman orator Seneca condoned these practices as common sense. Stories of ancient Spartan infanticide tickled Adolf Hitler's fancy for this reason. But archaeologists and historians struggle to find evidence of this happening on a society-wide scale. Of course, royalty and nobility of all stripes practiced some version of mate selection for centuries. Inbreeding with too-close kin occurred as a result. That "controlled breeding" probably resulted in the expression of otherwise rare hereditary diseases, hemophilia most notoriously. In the year 506, a Christian council of bishops at Agde (a town now in southern France) banned marriages between close family members, but not necessarily because of any hope to improve the overall human stock. It's hard to call any of these sporadic examples earnest attempts at following the human breeding advice of the ancients. Even among Plato devotees down the ages we find no concerted attempts to put into practice recommendations contained in book five of *Republic*. Then, in the last third of the nineteenth century, something changed.

> "We put down mad dogs; we kill the wild, untamed ox; we use the knife on sick sheep to stop their infecting the flock; we destroy abnormal offspring at birth; children, too, if they are born weak or deformed, we drown. Yet this is not the work of anger, but of reason: to separate the sound from the worthless."
> —Seneca, "On Anger," Book 1, 15.2 (c. 50 CE)[7]

About 2,300 years after Plato, a religious community in the US put selective breeding of humans into practice. In the Bible Commune in Oneida, New York, a theology student from Yale University and son of a US Congressman, John Humphrey Noyes, organized a selective breeding program he called "stirpiculture." (*Stirp* meaning "lineage" or "root" in Latin.) He had read his Plato, his Theognis, even his Darwin, alongside Bakewell livestock breeding manuals and Sunday School lessons. Noyes came to believe that humans were determined by the inborn, essential biological traits of our parents. It was right there in Genesis, where God created "kinds" and told them to make more of themselves. Noyes also inferred from Darwin's *On the Origin of Species* that, with careful selection, organisms could be primed to survive even in hostile environments. Humans could employ this knowledge for the glory of God and the betterment of humanity, Noyes and his Bible communists insisted. We could create healthier, happier children able to survive the wilds of the modern world using the biological rules God set up and Darwin discovered—if only we could be disciplined enough.

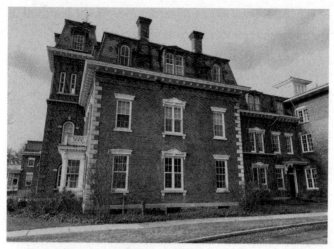

During the 1870s, John H. Noyes's Bible communists conducted a
sustained eugenics experiment in their Oneida, New York, compound.

From 1869 to 1879, one hundred men and women, almost
a third of the whole Oneida Commune, voluntarily submitted
to a selection process by a half dozen women and a half dozen
men. This committee of religious elders rigorously and prayer-
fully made selections based on spiritual, intellectual, moral,
and physical traits, in that order. Over the next decade, forty-
one mothers from the ages of twenty to forty-two conceived
to bear sixty-two children, fifty-eight of whom lived past age
three and fifty-two well into middle age. Given the standards
of the day, their offspring—"stirpicults," they were sometimes
called—remained a remarkably healthy, well-adjusted bunch.
When, in the 1920s, Dr. Hilda H. Noyes, one of the original
Oneida stirpicults and one of the first female MDs in the
history of New York state, conducted a statistical survey of
her fellow stirpicults, her findings (mainly about health and
longevity) seemed to demonstrate that controlled human
breeding—eugenics—could be overwhelmingly successful.[8]

By the late nineteenth century, even an American presidential candidate publicly advocated stirpiculture. Victoria Woodhull, a passionate advocate for women's rights, proclaimed during her campaign for president in 1872 that women should be able to exercise their constitutional and natural rights to couple and mate with whoever they wanted for as long or as short as they wanted. Women should be allowed to freely choose, Woodhull insisted, because only women could properly select traits that would make society better looking, healthier, stronger, more courageous, and more righteous. Animal breeders could build bigger, softer, tougher, or more compliant stock. Agriculturalists in the nineteenth century had already shown how much more yield humans could squeeze out of corn, cows, cotton, and wheat, given intentional scientific breeding practices. What was preventing the same in humans?

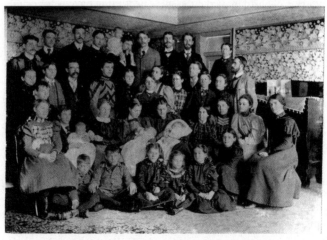

"Stirpicults": twelve healthy offspring of the Oneida eugenics experiments, 1892

Even after losing the election to the incumbent, Ulysses S. Grant, Woodhull blasted her message that the fate of humans was just as biologically determined as plants and animals at lecture after lecture around the North American speaking circuit. Then she did the same in her new home, the United Kingdom. Given biological determinism, Woodhull said, the responsibility of humanity couldn't be clearer: only the fit should have children.

> "Thou shalt not marry when malformed or diseased.
>
> Thou shalt not produce His image in ignorance.
>
> Thou shalt not defile His Temple!"
> —Victoria Woodhull, "Stirpiculture; or, the Scientific Propagation of the Human Race"[9]

From Woodhull's perspective, even Queen Victoria's once-pristine, well-managed cities were becoming havens for crime, poverty, alcoholism, and teeming hordes of the diseased. What did modern urbanites and their governments typically do with these sorts? Those fools preached charity. They cared for the mentally ill in institutions. They coddled. Biology taught that this sort of kindness was stupid, weak, and self-defeating, Woodhull lectured. Other organisms would have exterminated these inborn tendencies to crime, alcoholism, promiscuity, and whatever maladaptive trait they found thriving among their fellows. And eventually, those remaining organisms would have become fitter. Humans, by contrast, "niced" ourselves into degeneration, into larger numbers of humans needing to be cared for. According to her, it was high time someone managed the fate of humanity so that future generations would finally progress, not simply collect the weak.

The Oneida Bible communists and Victoria Woodhull were but two examples of a rapidly growing interest in the late nineteenth century on both sides of the Atlantic in controlling human breeding. After centuries, the fears and hopes expressed by Theognis and Plato became better

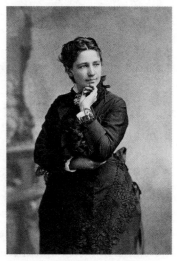

Victoria Woodhull, eugenicist for president, 1872

defined. They found cheerleaders. Physicians and politicians and psychologists fashioned whole terminologies to express these hopes and fears, names that seemed to convey scientific heft. And quietly, unbeknownst even to ardent supporters like Woodhull, some American medical men had arrived at an efficient process by which Theognis's ancient fears about sullying the blood could be addressed. But we'll get to that part of the story in a bit.

CHAPTER 2

Degenerates

What Victoria Woodhull captured in her speeches and publications was a deep-seated fear of the breeding potential of the unfit—the second ingredient, along with biological determinism, that was crucial to the rise of the eugenics movement in the twentieth century The worst sorts always seemed to have more babies than the best sorts. And this fear that Woodhull so cogently and powerfully expressed in Victorian America and Britain propelled a new version of eugenics.

Unlike the ancients, Theognis and Plato, for instance—unlike even Oneida's prayerful selection and communal rearing of chosen stirpiculs in the 1870s—modern eugenics focused on *eliminating* the unfit as much as it did *promoting* the fit. By the mid-1800s, several decades before Francis Galton even coined the word "eugenics," physicians and scientists raised the alarm that degenerate humans were increasing in number disproportionately to the rest of the population. If someone didn't act fast, civilization itself would be drowned by the undesirable. It's this fear of the fecundity of the unwanted that distinguishes modern eugenics from its ancient predecessors.

Much of the fear of degeneration can be traced back to physicians and politicians in French-speaking Europe, men like Joseph Arthur de Gobineau, Adolphe Quêtelet, and

Bénédict Morel. Each emphasized different facets of the fear of degeneration, and together, their worries shaped not only the modern eugenics movement but the Holocaust that followed.

Count Gobineau

Count Joseph Arthur de Gobineau really wanted to be a Viking. The problem was, though, that little Scandinavian blood actually coursed through his veins. But he continued to insist he was descended from those weather-beaten raiders who had leaped off longboats to ravage Christianized France and settle on the Normandy Coast centuries earlier. He built a whole worldview around his false belief about his own family's Viking heritage. Unbelievably, this one man's insecurity was reflected in and amplified by the generational insecurities of many, many other men for decades, creating a whole movement fetishizing Scandinavians and their descendants. He and his followers called them "Aryans," a word borrowed from the Sanskrit for "noble," to identify the best branch of the superior white race.

Gobineau cut his teeth as a research assistant for the illustrious Alexis de Tocqueville (famous for his Andrew Jackson-era *On Democracy in America*). After using that connection to launch an unsteady career as an aristocratic French diplomat, Gobineau wrote his misplaced ancestral pride into *Essai sur l'inégalité des races humaines* ("Essay on the Inequality of the Human Races," 1853–1855). He filled the four volumes with self-righteous pique that "bloody wars, the revolutions, and the breaking up of laws" as birthed by the American and French revolutions, and then the 1848 uprisings across Europe, reflected not the birth of freedom, but deep societal decay.[1] (In 1848, his own family's aristocratic worth had been depressed, as well—likely the more immediate trigger for his work.[2])

According to Gobineau, broad societal decay had a particular cause, one that he claimed was repeated through centuries of world history. In his imaginary chronicle, millennia ago, an original Aryan race responsible for "everything great, noble, and fruitful in the

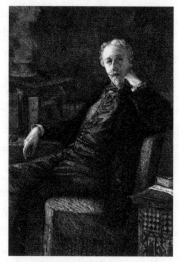

Count J. A. de Gobineau did the most to jump-start fears of racial degeneration.

works of man on this earth, in science, art, and civilization" spread across central Asia and into Europe pumping these regions full of *élan vital*, vital force, as they fought and settled and sculpted great philosophy and created great art and so on.[3] These original Aryans bore the "ten civilizations" that had structured the entirety of human history: the light-skinned Indians, pharaonic Egyptians, sea-faring Phoenicians, philosophic Greeks, conquering Romans, "white" Chinese, then "Germanic races"—including his mythologized Vikings—and, finally, the three empires in pre-Columbian America (Cahokia mound builders, Inca, and Aztecs).[4] Along their merry and bloody way, however, this superior Aryan race also interbred with the darker-skinned locals, descendants of either the original "Black" or the original "Yellow" races.

Apparently, however, there could be only so much of that vital force to go around. According to Gobineau, each generation that didn't inbreed with other Aryans dissipated their superior vital force. As the pure Aryan stock became more polluted by other races, rebellions, wars, and various types of collapses resulted. France itself was already degenerating. Inferior shorter and darker peasants—"nigridized" or "semitized," in Gobineau's terminology—intermingled with superior Aryan "Nordics" across Europe. The nefarious end would come when all those colors bled into one. He believed race mixing would ultimately drag down civilization itself.

Eventually, Gobineau traveled to many of the nations and regions bemoaned in his book—Teheran in what was then Persia; Athens, Greece; and Rio de Janeiro, Brazil—and in every case he believed he saw the degeneration through racial intermixing already well on its way. When he returned to France in 1870 to witness a military defeat by the Prussians, he triumphantly proclaimed his racist views vindicated in *Ce qui est arrivé à la France en 1870* ("What Happened to France in 1870")—race mixing led to France's defeat by the Germans, who possessed more pure Aryan blood.

Gobineau focused on fear, harnessed handwringing, and, like a prism, separated out the colors responsible for the looming demise of civilization—which was certainly lesser races. Intermingling Aryans with those lesser races dragged the whole system down because each race was biologically destined, determined, and carried some pure essence. Mixing those determined, essential races with the others would cause the degeneration of everything; and the unraveling may already have been underway.

Fear of race mixing: It's an underappreciated point. As we

will see later, the eugenics movement of the twentieth century seemed to take its cues from "family studies" of fictionalized clans in impoverished rural white America—the Jukes, Kallikaks, and many others—so-called white trash.[5] Some commentators have missed that this institutionalized eugenics was deeply connected to racial discrimination, which is understandable. After all, eugenics happened to Appalachian

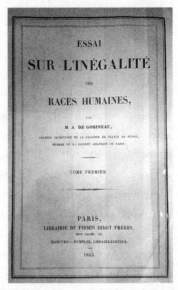

Gobineau's extremely influential Essai sur l'inégalité des races humaines

whites, to the white mentally ill in the northern half of the US, to white Germans in Germany—how could eugenics possibly be *racist*? Yet those nineteenth- and twentieth-century eugenics studies of impoverished whites were bolted onto an underlying speculation about racialized societal degeneration that emerged from European intellectuals like Gobineau. The degeneration narrative was, from Gobineau onward, tightly intertwined with anti-Black and anti-Brown, pro-Aryan and pro-Nordic racial hierarchies. It wasn't always expressed in a bigoted way, of course. But the downward spiral was always connected somehow to too many of a dark *them* and not enough of a light *us*. When "Gobineau Societies" championing Naziism emerged across Europe in the aftermath of World War I, they made the explicit connection that eugenically cleaning the white race was a means to continue dominating non-white races.

Bénédict Morel

Gobineau wasn't alone in his fear of degeneration. Around the same time, the French-trained psychiatrist Bénédict Augustin Morel (1809–1873), director of the Asile d'Aliénés de Saint-Yon (the Saint-Yon Insane Asylum) in Rouen, Normandy, recognized a disturbing trend. Heads were changing; brains were shrinking.[6] But he disagreed with the essentialism, the biological determinism, of Gobineau. Morel blamed degeneration on the modern city. With the growth of industry, urban environments squeezed the populace both metaphorically and literally, Morel conjectured. He saw the first disturbing sign of a rapidly changing environment in a wave of degenerate children. But he stressed that race mixing did not cause degeneration. Degeneration occurred because of the stresses of modern life.[7]

But even if Morel began in opposition to some of the fundamentals of eugenics, his work ended up supporting it. As Morel traveled to visit asylums and collect evidence across Europe, he began to notice that though raised by different parents in different nations, in different environments, and in different contexts, the mentally ill showed more similarities than not. Were these deviations from normal revealing "hereditary predispositions" visible in the head?[8] This was when Morel encountered the writing of the famed Belgian mathematician Adolphe Quêtelet.[9]

Having made a name for himself through his innovations in addressing astronomical error, Quêtelet quickly turned toward examining *social* "error." In 1834, Quêtelet witnessed a collection full of numerous deformed heads of ne'er-do-wells gleaned from hundreds of inmates in the mental asylums of Charenton, Bicêtre, and La Salpétrière, around Paris.[10] Quêtelet saw a pattern in the structure of the heads. In a breakthrough book published less than a year later, *Sur l'homme et le développement de ses facultés, ou essai de physique sociale* ("On Man and the Development of His Faculties; or, an Essay on Social Physics [Science]," 1835), Quêtelet stressed that alongside normal or "average" individuals there existed a substantial number who did not qualify as normal.[11] And here's the crucial takeaway, thought Quêtelet: It is from this number that most crime originates. He called them "monstrosit[ies]."[12] And their numbers were creeping steadily upward.[13]

From his place at Saint-Yon, Morel poured over Quêtelet's account. It rang true, given Morel's own experiences: The mentally unsound *were* growing more and more common. Asylums filled across Europe and America. And the worst part was the news that mentally degenerated individuals also carried a propensity for crime. Quêtelet claimed that "moral illnesses are like physical illnesses: some of them are contagious, some of them are epidemic, some others are hereditary."[14] Indeed, Morel noted statistics that crime was rising in parallel to the trend in asylum populations. Property crime, surely, but violence against persons as well. And suicides. And all manner of nasty behaviors that made society less safe, less pleasant. It also affected the national defense; the French military reported that recruits appeared in notably worse condition than in the past. Government ministers were alarmed, physicians were alarmed, police were alarmed, even religious figures were alarmed. Society showed every sign of decay and degeneration.

Maybe it could be arrested through decreasing filth, increasing food supplies, rationalizing cities, and taming industrialism. But Morel hesitated. If Quêtelet was right, were the mentally degenerate actually different *sorts* of humans, "pathological deviants" from the ordinary type? If so, then, unable to perform their tasks in society, degenerates became true burdens. Morel had read Lamarck and the other evolutionists. He knew that certain characteristics once acquired could be passed on from generation to generation. Some would pass on their degenerate traits to their offspring.[15] Alcoholism seemed to be hereditary.[16] Maybe other degenerate traits were too. Given a sufficient number, society as a whole would begin to crumble.

So, though it's true that Morel disavowed Gobineau's racism, he merely transformed a degeneration concept already freighted with plenty of racism into something scientific, connected with precise data, with heads and skulls and statistics. This is the theory that lasted, one of the key ingredients of modern eugenics: Civilization itself is decaying by allowing essentially degenerate individuals to roam free, commit crimes, and reproduce—increasing their future numbers.

In France, the notion stuck. During the Franco-Prussian War in the early 1870s, a pamphlet floated around Paris titled "La France dégénerée" that basically repeated Morel.

> "[We French are becoming] a degraded and dangerous populace, the downgraded, the perverted, the shameless, the deranged of all kinds, ... [visible in] the human scum that infests the capitals, in the epileptic and scrofulous scoundrel who, heir to stale blood and

> damaged by his own misconduct, imports degenera-
> tion and imbecility into civilization, maddens [civi-
> lization] with . . . backward instincts, and his badly
> constructed brain."
>
> —Anonymous, *La France dégénerée*[17]

A decade later, Charles Féré, a physician at the Bicêtre
Asylum in Paris, followed up on these fears with much more
data. In *Dégénérescence et criminalité* ("Degeneracy and Criminality," 1888), he repeated findings from the newly invented
myograph, which measured nervous excitement and reaction times. It demonstrated to Féré that, while some kinds of
degenerates would of course react too slowly, others showed
surprising dexterity—the kind that would benefit, say, thieves,
burglars, and murderers. And from there, degeneration fears
permeated popular novels in France and beyond.

The influential French novelist Émile Zola read Féré and
found this anxiety about degeneration prescient. He anchored
the twenty novels of his Rougon-Macquart series, including
masterpieces like *Germinal* (1885) and *La Bête humaine* ("The
Human Beast," 1890), to Morelian concepts of hereditary
degeneration. The British writer, criminal anthropologist,
and eventual sexologist Henry Havelock Ellis translated *Germinal* into English in 1894. Soon thereafter, Ellis channeled
Zola's fears of degeneration into his own advocacy for eugenics. Zola's handwringing over degeneration also rubbed off on
Fyodor Dostoyevsky, the "Shakespeare of the Russian novel."[18]

These culture-defining authors demonstrate that degeneration was no abstruse theory held by marginalized cranks.
By the last two decades of the nineteenth century, it was easy
enough to show proper scientific data supporting exactly

what Gobineau, Morel, and Quêtelet had feared a generation earlier: a degenerated populace was filling Europe's cities like silent, cancerous cells. And soon "degeneration" meant not only disease but violent crime.

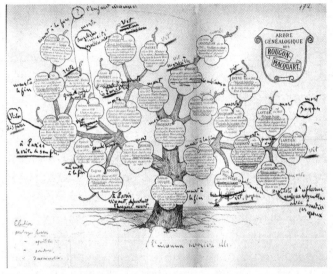

This tree graphically represents the fear of hereditary taint among the characters in Zola's celebrated Rougon-Macquart series. The members of the family further from the noble trunk increasingly exhibit the degenerative traits that Gobineau, Morel, and Quêtelet had warned about decades earlier.

CHAPTER 3

Natural-Born Criminals

By the late 1800s, increasing numbers of scientific and medical professionals agreed with their French colleagues that all sorts of negative behaviors, including alcoholism, violence, and crime, derived from traits locked in the individual by virtue of hidden biological essences passed on from their parents. Moral sickness, like physical illness, came down to biological essences. And if something wasn't done soon, the fecund unfit would overwhelm the fit and society would degenerate.

Still, these concerns seemed largely theoretical and confined to a select few. The third ingredient that led to twentieth-century eugenics was the apparent confirmation from hard biological evidence that degeneration was occurring. From head-bump-reading phrenology (the study of the shape and size of the cranium to indicate internal intellectual and personality traits) sprang this third ingredient: "criminal anthropology," the scientific hunt for telltale markers of temperament that would one day lead to criminal behavior—*pre*-crime written into the flesh. Criminal anthropologists across the globe looked for the stigmata of degeneration in a jutting jaw or a too-narrow bridge of the nose, physical signs these medical men warned would erupt into criminality. The most dangerous marks, the anthropologists warned, were "atavisms," or throwbacks, some trait from ages past that clung just under the surface, hidden but ready to reemerge—the savage beast concealed within.

Particulate inheritance + Biological determinism

↓

Scientific racism + Degeneration

↓

Atavism + Criminal anthropology

↓

EUGENICS

Some contemporary scholars blame this belief of partially buried atavistic bestiality on Charles Darwin's natural selection, Gregor Mendel's genetics, or Sigmund Freud's psychotherapy. But, in truth, this fascination with the reappearance of buried ancestral traits had already appeared a century earlier. In the mid-1700s, the French philosopher and physiologist Pierre-Louis Moreau de Maupertuis recorded cases of families with polydactyly (having more than five fingers or toes) that seemed to skip generations and concluded that these biological mistakes represented the return of deep ancestral traits. "Amazing," thought Maupertuis, yet "too frequent to be considered as doubtful."[1] Some ancestral traits persisted a very long time, revealing lines of descent *without* modification.

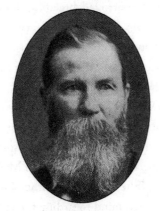

E. P. Fowler, supposedly not a phrenologist like his brothers

By the 1870s, works such as Charles Darwin's

The Descent of Man and Selection in Relation to Sex (1871) and *The Expression of the Emotions in Man and Animals* (1872) finally convinced many scientists that the human mind was also a product of descent with modification. Then, these new criminal anthropologists and their physician fellow travelers had a bit of an "aha moment." Mental features were precisely the sorts of differences where a Maupertuisan interpretation—a throwback to a more "primitive" trait—perhaps associated with a primitive (*read*: non-white) race—would be most obvious. Still, how much could anyone *demonstrate* this difference physiologically?

Dissecting Heads

Edward Payson Fowler was the younger half brother of Lorenzo and Orson Fowler, New York City's most famous phrenologists. You've likely seen one of the Fowlers' white phrenological busts in an antique shop. All three Fowler brothers lived with their sister, Charlotte Fowler Wells, a prolific publisher against tobacco and for vegetarianism, feminism, and controlled breeding. Edward used family connections to join Louis Pasteur in the 1870s at the height of Pasteur's influence. Fowler was at Pasteur's side for the world-changing bacteriology that convinced the medical community of germ theory—invisible biological essences could cause sickness. Once back in New York, Fowler became a respected fixture of the New York medical community, raising money for the founding of New York Hospital and serving as president of the New York Academy of Medicine for over twenty years.[2]

In 1875, his half brother, Lorenzo Fowler, an expert on the human mind regarding the culpability of criminals, weighed in. "If it can be proved that a man has no 'moral sense,'" speculated Lorenzo, "he should be recognized as being unfit . . . and should be confined to an institution." If, he suggested, we admitted that there were men "lower than the savage" who walked among us but, because of our own feelings of charity about their mental illnesses, we did not punish them, crime would overwhelm our cities.[3]

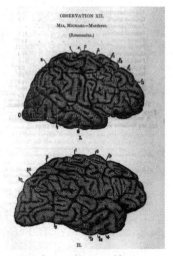

The dissected criminal brain, according to degeneration theorists

E. P. Fowler echoed his half brother in an 1880 academic article "Are the Brains of Criminals Anatomical Perversions?" to which he answered his own question with an unequivocal *yes*. Brains of "constitutional" criminals, E. P. Fowler insisted, looked more like the brains of those of a "primitive race."[4] A year later, in 1881, he translated and popularized a particularly inspirational European text outlining the precise nature of those "anatomical perversions" in *Anatomical Studies Upon Brains of Criminals* by Viennese neurosurgeon Moritz Benedikt.

For his contribution to, as he put it, a "Natural History of Crime," Benedikt dissected the brains of twelve criminals and found that the fissures exhibited by criminal brains cut far deeper and connected with one another in places where they would remain separated in comparison to a "normal" brain. Destiny written in folds of gray matter. If only more police, more wardens, and more psychologists who worked with criminals could see the degree to which the "defective, atypically-constructed brain" determined the habitual criminal, then we could forge a more just and humane society.[5]

E. P. Fowler translated Benedikt's entire study from German into English for a simple reason: America was terrible at rehabilitating criminals.[6] It would be better for the criminal and for society, Fowler insisted, to keep defectives from being free in the first place. And all the better if you could see which people were defective *before* they committed crimes. This is where criminal anthropology could really do some good. *Anthropology*. Not phrenology. Not craniometry. Bumps and creases *in* the brain—not mere bumps and creases on the scalp—which translate to features visible *on* the face and neck. His ideas were completely different from his half brothers' pseudoscientific phrenology, his medical supporters claimed, and much more scientific than his sister's writings against the dangers of red meat, alcohol swilling, and cigar smoking. *This* Fowler's kind of biological determinism was real science.

Increasingly, prison wardens bought it. They agreed that criminality was hardwired in the brain, and by the 1880s you could read it in their annual reports.[7] According to the progressive Eastern State Penitentiary inspectors: "There is an inherited trait or taint in many, which may possibly lead to the commission of crimes, a motor, as it were, that unconsciously impels those who suffer from this hereditary taint, to become criminals."[8] By the 1890s, terms such as "inherent depravity," "mental disease," and "hereditary crime-cause" appeared more and more often in the records of new inmates filling their prison.

Insane in the Membrane

A particularly significant pivot point in the acceptance of criminal anthropology in the US occurred in 1881. Charles Guiteau, a former member of the Oneida Bible Commune (but not a stirpicult), assassinated President James Garfield. Guiteau's attorney then unsuccessfully attempted an insanity defense. The whole incident whet the nation's appetite for salacious true-crime stories. And, what's more, the assassin's case defined what was at stake with regard to fears of degeneration and hereditary crime more sharply than any previous medical publication. Not surprisingly, over the 1880s, American medical journals, newsletters, and magazines swung palpably in their tone and coverage toward locating, identifying, charting, classifying, and explaining hereditary taint and, specifically, the hereditary criminal.

Guiteau's performance in the courtroom undoubtedly led many more medical workers to consider criminality just one more defect of the more broadly mentally ill. He hooted displeasure, grandstanded, cackled inappropriately, gesticulated wildly, and interrupted council, witness, and judge indiscriminately throughout the trial. Despite many warnings that he would be punished for his outbursts, Guiteau seemed unable to control himself. The defense then used this very behavior to underscore its insanity defense. But the assassin also revealed a good deal of cleverness; he was not so obviously mentally impaired that he lacked reasoning power.[9] He claimed God told him to assassinate the president, which, by nineteenth-century standards, was a kind of heresy. And, anyway, for the murder of the nation's symbolic leader, the American public wanted blood.

After executioners marched Guiteau to the gallows, neurologists swooped in to cut open his brain. The alienist (an

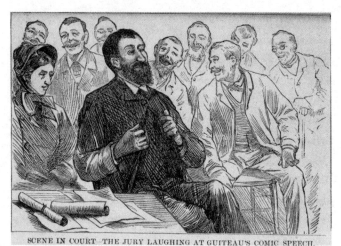

SCENE IN COURT—THE JURY LAUGHING AT GUITEAU'S COMIC SPEECH.

Charles Guiteau's performance during trial—and later, his brain, after he was executed—became an early test of the criminal insanity concept and legal defense.

early term for psychiatrist) Charles Karsner Mills, dubbed the "dean of American neurology" from his post at the University of Pennsylvania, dove in to the criminal anthropology conversation by carefully examining Guiteau's gray matter. "Criminality from a purely scientific standpoint," was what Mills promised, and Dr. Mills's "Mental Disorders: Reflections on Criminal Lunacy, with Remarks on the Case of Guiteau" (1882) reported that the assassin's brain indeed showed hereditary defects.[10] By the time he was done dissecting Guiteau's brain, Mills had convinced many of his most prestigious colleagues in the American neurological community that inherited criminal brains made criminals.[11]

Lombroso's Delayed Effect

In this fevered environment, it was much too easy for American medical professionals, law enforcement, and the legal system itself to wield this concept of hereditary taint visible in the brain. Lingering support for Fowler phrenology then led to an even sloppier version of criminal anthropology, promoted by the Italian criminologist Cesare Lombroso.

Too often, modern criminal justice scholars portray the work of Lombroso as revolutionary for American criminal theorists. But Lombroso's celebrated formation of the criminal anthropology did not crash like a wave over American criminology after he penned his famous *L'Uomo delinquente studiato in rapporto all'antropologia, alla medicina legale ed alla discipline carcerarie* ("The Criminal Man Studied in Relation to Anthropology, Forensics, and Penology") in 1876. It's important to point this out because nothing could be further from the truth. Instead, Lombroso's prejudices about the physical appearance, or physiognomy, and more specialized conversations about brains and skulls already circulating around the US, such as those promoted by physicians like E. P. Fowler, merged. Then they metastasized silently in the American medical community. By the mid-1880s, the Lombrosian prejudices embedded within both Italian and American criminal anthropology absorbed adjacent fields in science and birthed the nascent discipline of jail and prison management—what we now call criminal justice.

According to Lombroso and his followers, tattooing, scarring, and physical deformities represented the stigmata of moral deficiency, sexual deviance, homosexuality, and potential criminality. In other words, Lombroso, who reportedly displayed a Fowlerian phrenological bust on his desk, migrated the stigmata of phrenology from the bumpy head to the whole body.[12] Revisiting the notion of atavism, Lombroso saw the sins of even deep ancestors called forth once again in the bodies of their descendants.

In the mid-1860s, Lombroso published two books on the hereditary persistence of behavioral traits. The more famous of the two, *Genio e follia* ("Genius and Madness," 1864), became forever ensconced as an axiom: the uncomfortable proximity of genius to insanity. Yet it was in *L'uomo bianco e l'uomo di colore* ("The

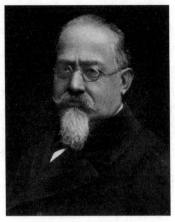

Cesare Lombroso

White Man and the Black Man," 1871)—a book perhaps wisely left untranslated into English—that Lombroso revealed his deeper project. Charles Darwin wrestled with race in *Descent of Man* (1871), deciding that female preference must be largely responsible for the persistence of many racial traits in humans that seemed to confer no direct survival benefit. Lombroso, at the same moment, stressed the permanent primitiveness of the dark-skinned by adding his observations and analogies to the old scientific racism of Gobineau, among others. Crania, Lombroso confidently parroted in *L'uomo bianco e l'uomo di colore*, revealed to him that whites would never need "bow their foreheads" to any other race.[13]

Blunt Aryan superiority and anti-Blackness based on rehashing older scientific racist work also permeated Lombroso's most famous work, *The Criminal Man* (1876). Though it would not be translated into English until the twentieth century, florid Lombrosian descriptions of hereditary criminals, guided by the "ferocious instincts of primitive humanity and the inferior animals," seeped into almost all expressions of criminal anthropology in the late nineteenth century.[14] Given the degree to which they published these views openly, we have to conclude that turn-of-the-century medical men and prison professionals believed these things as a matter of course.

Charles Mills (the "dean of American neurology") continued publishing his brain studies widely after his work on Guiteau's brain, and they only became more sophisticated. In his June 1886 presidential address to the American Neurological Association, for instance, the eminent brain surgeon announced his study of comparative cerebral topography at a level surpassing even Benedikt or Lombroso. In his (according to him) very scientific address, he stated his head collection included a grab bag of the degenerated: a "delusional lunatic"—a criminal whose life was nothing more than a "sickening tale of lust and violence," a "feeble-minded youth," an epileptic, a Chinese "coolie," and "Ford, an ignorant negro." The brains of these figures, claimed Mills, appeared

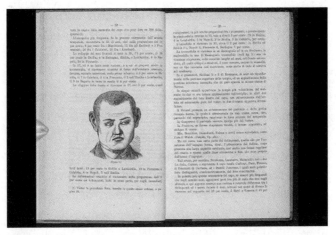

One of Lombroso's depictions of the criminal visage (1876)

malformed, almost fetal, with development arrested, throwbacks from a more primitive time. Knowing the way that the deep, dark, savage past had the ability to erupt like magma through fissures in the long-laid strata of heredity, Mills thought—like Lombroso, and like Maupertuis almost two centuries earlier—that responsibility fell to tough-minded scientists like him to warn and defend society from hereditary taint lodged in cerebral fissures and gyres of "paranoiacs, criminals, idiots, and negroes."[15] The menace of the unfit persisted from parent to child to grandchild to great-grandchild, sapping society's strength.

Science to Sci-Fi

Increasing numbers of reformers, criminologists, and others intrigued by criminal anthropology in the 1880s and 1890s followed Mills, Fowler, and Lombroso in asserting that crime was a result of a biological defect. According to them, one could see the predilection to sin, to violate, on the face and the head. But you could see it in other ways too. The highly trained medical professionals said congenital criminals favored tattoos. Their brow ridges protruded. An ape-like jaw jutted. Anyone might see the signs, if only they knew what to look for.

Unsurprisingly, some of this percolated into pop culture. Bram Stoker told us in 1897 that Count Dracula would have been designated as being of the "criminal type" by Lombroso, given his unibrow, hawkish nose, protruding teeth, and other obvious physiognomic indicators.[16] And the Victorian icon Dr. Jekyll's alter ego, Mr. Hyde, reeks of the ape-like Lombrosian atavistic criminal.[17] Arthur Conan Doyle swam in these literary waters too. He placed Sherlock Holmes only below the great

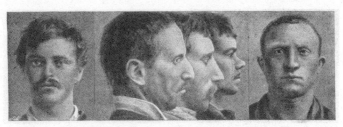

Alphonse Bertillon's policing through criminal anthropology: The "mug shot" becomes the standard tool of criminal diagnostics.

(and nonfictional) Alphonse Bertillon for detective genius. Bertillon made criminal anthropology practical.

The French detective Alphonse Bertillon used criminal anthropology to revolutionize policing in Paris. The "Bertillon system" captured fore and side photographs of criminals' heads—the now classic mug shot (first proposed, ironically, by Sir Francis Galton, only to be superseded by his own advocacy for criminal fingerprinting). Bertillon combined the photographs with careful cranial measurements and hair- and eye-color indexing.

Here is a telling moment. Early in the twentieth century, new experts on the Continent challenged the need for Bertillon's identification system, since by then fingerprinting had become ubiquitous and was thought to be more reliable for criminal identification. But Detective Bertillon himself fought against dropping the head measuring system, in part because it was incredibly accurate for identification. But he also fought its departure because criminal photography (*portrait parle*), which grouped hair, eye, and skin colors, tattoos, nose shapes, and peculiar skull characteristics, was never exclusively about *identification* alone. With a robust criminal database, Bertillon could continue to hunt for "criminal *propensities*." Indeed, it was for these reasons—not just identification of suspects but the hope of uncovering hereditary taint and arresting societal degeneration—that American police departments adopted the Bertillon mug shot system, even as it died out in Europe.[18]

A few acknowledged just how closely criminal anthropology resembled pseudoscientific phrenology. But not many. Instead, they published real, peer-reviewed, scientific articles showing its use. Dozens at first. Then scores. From London and Paris and Berlin. And then from Boston to Charleston, Chicago to New Orleans. Physicians and prison reformers, moralists and uplifters, then preachers and detectives and police officers. They spilled forth in weekly digests and annual reports and conference papers and debates at local gatherings and national publications in magazines and newspapers. Their presentations ranged from speculative ("Crime: Its Physiology and Pathenogenesis. How Far Can Medical Men Aid in Its Prevention?") to concrete ("Criminals the Product of Hereditary Degeneracy") to pragmatic ("The Coming Role of the Medical Profession in the Scientific Treatment of Crime and Criminals") to, frankly, *creepy* ("Criminality and Degeneracy; Its Treatment by Surgery and Hypnotism").[19]

Redeeming the Sin of Hereditary Taint

Something must be done, surgeons and wardens, police chiefs and politicians said. Criminal reformers wanted more humane treatment of criminals. And all seemed to agree on the unnecessary brutality of the justice system, especially in America. But they believed that addressing individual criminals directly would prove more effective than general, oblique, and costly alterations to schooling, training, hygiene, public infrastructure, and reducing social and economic inequality. How could they use the powers of science and medicine to halt the degenerative path society found itself on? How could they do so humanely, without the punitive violence so often meted out by the criminal justice system?

There were scientific ideas out there, floated by the English polymath Francis Galton in 1883: encourage the right sorts to outbreed the degenerate sorts. This is what Galton called "eugenics."

But American physicians also had other medical techniques closer at hand. Decades earlier, an outspoken physician from Texas popularized a medical method that provided the powerful with their own tools to mold future society more directly. Dr. Gideon Lincecum proclaimed that the best way to stop social degeneration was for physicians—men like him, to be more precise—to have the authority to eliminate unborn generations of the unfit. We must use the powers of science and medicine to limit the spread of negative traits from parent to child, Lincecum trumpeted. And had his "Lincecum Memorial" law passed in the 1850s or '60s, Texas would have become the first state to legalize sterilization—even coercive, compulsory castration—for criminals, alcoholics, political agitators, and other degenerates.

Lincecum's law didn't pass. Still, the next generation of physicians parroted him. In 1893, Texas physician F. E. Daniel proposed sterilizing insane criminals and homosexuals.[20] From Cincinnati to Chicago to New York, and from Virginia to Tennessee to Kansas, medical journals reveal that physicians already had begun sporadically employing a surgical fix for a whole host of—from their perspective—social illnesses, including sexual deviance. And gradually, the work of Francis Galton on hard heredity, under his label "eugenics," began to trickle into American medicine.

CHAPTER 4

From Sir Francis Galton
to Connecticut

Sir Francis Galton has long been deemed the "father of eugenics." But as you now know, this moniker is an oversimplification. He coined the word in 1883 and then lived long enough to see it become a special interest group with political clout in London. University College London then launched the first academic professorship in eugenics in his honor. In terms of real actions ensconcing eugenics in the fabric of societies, however, Galton can hardly be ranked as more than a figurehead. As we'll soon see, the first eugenics legislation was passed in Connecticut. The true "fathers of eugenics," then, would be the forgotten legislators who authored, introduced, and passed that bill in 1895.

Still, Galton deserves special attention, which I will give him here. His name is the first one we typically encounter in conventional histories of eugenics for a reason. It was Galton who wove together strands from statistics, biology, medicine, and the new field of sociology into a single, coherent story about who should be allowed to bear children and why. He began by reestablishing the ancient belief in biological essences that determine the fates of individuals, and perhaps even nations and racial groups. Just before he died, Galton saw the idea of all-powerful essences transformed into belief in hardened particles, shielded from the environment. He may even have heard them referred to by their new scientific name: "genes." Indeed, it was Galton more than anyone who began the process of making *biological* determinism into *genetic* determinism.[1] In other words, when we look to the *ideas* half of the eugenics story, Galton is the one who took the angst over degeneration

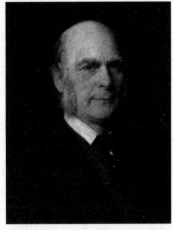

Sir Francis Galton is often labeled the "father of eugenics," though that's only true if we focus on scientific ideas and not medical practices.

from Gobineau onward, put a mathematical sheen on it, and trotted it out as cutting-edge biological research.

Given the other figures we've already encountered who decried societal decay and promoted controlled human breeding, how is it that Galton became the individual singled out as the "father of eugenics"? To answer that, we must go back decades before Galton coined "eugenics" in 1883, to the years he fashioned a particular exacting and, in the end, very influential scientific persona.

The real father-of-eugenics Galton story begins in the 1870s. And it starts with rabbits. Or, rather, the blood of one color of rabbit transfused into another one again and again and again. The bodies and blood of transfused rabbits piled up, becoming quite a nuisance to the zookeepers. And the whole thing was sort of Charles Darwin's fault.

This merits some explanation.

Darwin's Soft Inheritance Problem

To explain the resemblance of living things both to long-buried fossils and to each other, Darwin's *On the Origin of Species* (1859) convinced many naturalists of the importance of shared ancestry—common descent, in other words. But scientists worried that Darwin's whole story of evolution left out two key components. Why were children like their parents (inheritance)? And why were they not *exactly* like their siblings (variation)? Aside from saying "plants and animals vary," what physical mechanism could Darwin provide to fill in these twin gaps in his otherwise solid idea about differential survival and reproduction (i.e., natural selection)? For some critics, the absence of a biological mechanism made Darwin's whole scheme feel far too speculative.

Darwin tried to meet the criticisms, of course. By the mid-1860s, he had gathered enough material on rabbits and orchids and pigeons and dogs and livestock to publish the first volume of his Big Project: *The Variation of Animals and Plants Under Domestication* (1868). Darwin tucked his single mechanism, a silver bullet to explain both variation and inheritance, way in the back of the second volume. "Pangenesis," he called it. He made sure to label it merely a "provisional hypothesis," as Darwin seemed concerned about how scientific colleagues would receive it.[2] Spoiler alert: *They cringed*.

For fifty pages of *Variation*, Darwin speculated that particles called "gemmules," scattered throughout the body, swelled and swelled during development until they became the visible parts of an organism. Something akin to pomegranate seeds growing into organs and limbs, I suppose. Of course, those slowly swelling gemmules received various inputs throughout their existences, bumps and nicks and scratches and scars, mostly. Some of those would be direct, even traumatic, injuries. Some of these gemmules, now altered through the process of being kicked around by life for a while, separated from the others and gathered in the sex cells. From there they had a chance to transmit their combined inherited and directly acquired characteristics to the next generation. So, from Darwin's perspective, the biological fact of variation, which was crucial for his concept of natural selection, emerged as little parcels of inheritance, scuffed up a bit, then delivered to the next generation. (Yes, in case you picked up on it, it makes Darwin's version of evolution seem a lot more like Jean-Baptiste Lamarck's than we care to admit.)

Darwin was right to worry about how his theory would be received. Pangenesis was an idea too old and out of style by the 1860s to even call it retro.[3] Even his supporters remained

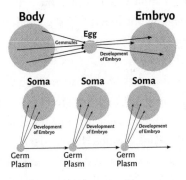

According to Charles Darwin's pangenesis theory, every part of the body emits tiny particles, or gemmules, that migrate to the gonads and contribute to the fertilized egg and sperm to create the next generation. But gemmules are open to environmental inputs. In the "germ" theory of inheritance that undergirds twentieth-century genetics, by contrast, hereditary material is confined to the germs (genes) in the gonads. Body parts (soma) develop afresh in each generation from the germ plasm and are not open to change through the environment. Galton supported germ plasm theory against his cousin's pangenesis.

skeptical. Though Darwin promised to "try to persuade myself not to publish," three years later, there pangenesis sat, splayed out in print for everyone to gawk at.[4] His critics pounced. Had he *seen* a gemmule? Had anyone? The hypothesis of pangenesis felt threadbare.

Still, Darwin needed some hypothesis for how natural selection was possible. What was selected? Where else did variation come from? When it came to this inheritance of acquired characteristics stuff—the cause of variation, from which nature carefully selected to improve the race little by little—Darwin had to commit. He had no better explanation.

His cousin Francis Galton had other ideas.

Francis Galton's New Particulate Determinism

Severe, balding, hawk-nosed, stern (the man seemed incapable of cracking a smile), Galton had been quietly collecting scientific credentials for himself in the application of statistics to natural phenomenon. His *Meteorographica* (1863) transformed the way we look at weather; his maps are the great-great-grandparents of your smartphone's weather app. Galton self-financed his own voyage into southwest Africa in the 1850s, on which he got to name the chunks of land he traversed, Willy Wonka–esque "Damaraland" and "Ovampoland." He penned a widely read book out of the adventure, *Narrative of an Explorer in Tropical South Africa* (1853). It was no *Voyage of the Beagle*, perhaps, but it was pretty good. Cousin Charles liked it.[5]

Soon, Galton turned his gaze toward that notion of inheritance himself. Just like big zones of high and low barometric pressure floating across maps, Galton noticed a tendency for talent to blow through family lines. Not surprisingly, he located a jet stream of talent in his own tightly integrated Galton-Darwin-Wedgwood family. He spent about a year tracing lineages and, in 1864 and 1865, published the two-part essay "Hereditary Talent and Character." The character he traced was greatness itself. Galton had used Phillips's *The Million of Facts*, the Wikipedia of its day, to hunt the lineages of around three hundred learned British men. In what we might now consider a "big data" project, Galton calculated that one was much more likely to be eminent if one had an eminent man in one's family tree.[6] Greatness, in other words, ran through the right sorts of families—families like his. (If Galton's conclusions seem painfully self-serving to us, take comfort in the fact that they seemed that way to Galton's peers as well. Few took notice of his work, initially.)

Three years and a nervous breakdown later, Galton went at it again. *Hereditary Genius: An Inquiry Into Its Laws and Consequences* (1869) assayed the lineages of judges, statesmen, poets, scientists, painters, and other elites (even "wrestlers of the north country") to assert that in every case, nature trumped nurture.[7] *That's* what he meant. But even as this book wasn't a hit, it planted a flag. Decades later, the British scientific community would rally around the importance of inheritance.[8] Darwin told Galton he liked it. But Darwin hadn't really read it closely. Only George Howard Darwin, the second Darwin son, had finished reading the book. Charles had missed Galton's main point—namely, that it was anti-Darwin.

> "I have no patience with the hypothesis occasionally expressed, and often implied, especially in tales written to teach children to be good, that babies are born pretty much alike, and that the sole agencies in

> creating differences between boy and boy, and man
> and man, are steady application and moral effort. It is
> in the most unqualified manner that I object to pre-
> tensions of natural equality."
> —Francis Galton, *Hereditary Genius: An Inquiry Into*
> *Its Laws and Consequences*[9]

Soft inheritance, environmentalism, acquired characteristics—whatever one called it, Galton opposed it. He wanted
to overturn those theories. He thought instead that traits
were *hard*, discrete particles. They passed on from parent to
child as if they were marbles, with almost no influence from
the outside world. They were solid batons in an intergenera-
tional relay race. You are an agglutination of *essences* passed
down from generation to generation; it's that old biological
determinism that Galton wanted to make great again. Darwin's pangenesis represented a weight on the wrong side of the
intellectual scales. Gemmules were too *soft*. They suggested
that the environment did matter—quite a lot, in fact. Galton
meant to fix that.

And now we get to the rabbits.

The Rabbit Experiments

"My dear Darwin, I wonder if you could help me," began Galton
in a December 1869 letter. Some "peculiar experiments" had just
popped into his head, ideas that spoke directly to Darwin's pangenesis chapter in *Variation*. In it, Darwin cited the experiences
of rabbit breeders, especially those who bred Angora albinos.
These are the pure white rabbits we envision emerging from a
black velvet top hat. Galton wanted some of those. And only

Darwin knew precisely where to get these exact specimens in large enough quantities.[10] Darwin may have sensed something was up, but he magnanimously made the suggestions and the personal connections, promising to help.

Throughout 1870, Francis Galton conducted infamous experiments to demonstrate that Darwin's theory of pangenesis was incorrect. Once he successfully bred the pure white Angora rabbits, he began transfusing their blood with those of rabbits with darker color coats. After transfusion, he had the rabbits breed only with those that shared their existing coat color: light with light, dark with dark. If Darwin's pangenesis theory was correct, the babies of transfused rabbits would sport coats a bit more like the blood-donor rabbits. Dark-furred parents would have babies with somewhat lighter fur or with spots of lightness; and the reverse would also be true. Pangenesis predicted that the gemmules, as particles of heredity, floated through the veins of the receiving parents and then on to their children, "mongrelizing" them, in Galton's terms, from their expected coloration. Pure Angora whiteness would be blemished.

For a bloody year and more, Galton transfused rabbit blood, successfully de-fibrinizing to prevent clotting, pumping larger and larger quantities into each rabbit, and reported to Darwin his findings. Then in March 1871, Galton rose to speak before the venerable Royal Society of London. His paper "Experiments in Pangenesis, by Breeding from Rabbits of a Pure Variety, into Whose Circulation Blood Taken from Other Varieties Had Previously Been Largely Transfused" spelled out all of his painstaking work. The first extensive test of Darwin's hypothesis was a resounding negative. *No pangenesis.*

Then, without a word about his results, which were just then circulating in scientific journals—Galton must have known Darwin would read them—Galton pleasantly sent some of the rabbit survivors to Darwin and his children to play with and enjoy over the Easter holiday.[11]

Indeed, Darwin found out. He dashed off a tense letter to *Nature* objecting that he had never said "blood" exactly. Gemmules could be just about anywhere in the body. Maybe they were in the nerves. In the publications of "water-cure" aficionados—and Darwin was an absolute devotee of the water cure, heading to the Malvern-area spas whenever he or his children felt really ill—the idea was widely believed that the shock of cold water, combined with plenty of imbibed pure water, would unplug the nerves, allowing them to flow. Darwin's protest may have come from a commitment to seeing the nerves as the conduits of pangenesis. In any case, Galton's rabbit experiments had missed the true fluid and, therefore, the true genius of pangenesis, said Darwin. Of course, Darwin neglected to mention that he had corresponded with Galton through the whole thing, and that Darwin knew all along Galton was testing blood.

Galton apologized, stating that all Darwin's references to "circulation" in *Variation* must have thrown him off. Because what systems, other than blood, circulate? His bending over backward to apologize to Darwin masked the fact that Galton's wet work from 1870 to 1871 set him concretely against all the soft heredity stuff that evolutionists from Lamarck to Darwin had peddled to an impressionable public. Hard deterministic "nature" clearly won out against soft "nurture"—this was what the rabbits had taught him.

Resolute, Galton floated two very public trial balloons advocating a more aggressive stance toward heredity and its impact upon society in 1873—after Darwin's *Descent of Man, and Selection in Relation to Sex* gripped naturalists with an *even softer* mechanism of inheritance, sexual selection, that would help explain problems like the origins of human races.

Galton's More Aggressive Applied Science

In Galton's first essay, titled "Hereditary Improvement," he proposed that in toxic British cities, only the most brutish people would thrive—like cockroaches, rats, and other vermin. The old, solid Anglo-Saxon racial stock, on the other hand, was already showing signs of degeneration, as Gobineau had warned. If not halted, the slide might look something like what happened to Ireland after the mid-century famine. The Irish were even more degenerate than ever before, he said; they were now a chapter in Galton's morality tale of how the replication of less desirable stock could physically and mentally drag a whole people down into savagery. If Britain could establish special castes composed of superior individuals within each ordinary class group, and encourage those individuals to have numerous, hearty, white, English-speaking children, they could reverse the slide toward barbarism brought on by filthy, undermanaged urbanization punctuated by the immigration of lesser races who intermarried with native stock.[12]

Galton saw an opportunity here. It was like the breeding of rabbits. First, he called it *not* eugenics but "viriculture"—encouraging only the Aryan race to breed exclusively. In truth, it was the Oneida Community's "stirpiculture" with a new prefix, and he surely knew it. At an important meeting of the Sociological Society of London in 1904 where Galton again championed his eugenics ideas, the literary icon H. G. Wells scolded Galton for not giving appropriate credit. "Stirpiculture" indicated John Humphrey Noyes's American experiment. Viriculture was a knockoff. Galton grumpily denied this.

For some cultures in some places, however, encouraging better breeding would not be enough. In Galton's second article from 1873, "Africa for the Chinese," he advocated genocide right on the pages of *The Times* of London. "The gain would be immense to the whole civilized world," stated Galton, "if we were to out-breed and finally displace the negro, as completely as the latter has displaced the aborigines of the West Indies."[13] As Galton saw it, the white-run British Empire should create a Chinese state in East Africa and physically move Chinese to live and work the land, just as the young US had attempted to do in Liberia on Africa's northwest coast decades earlier. The Africans would go extinct. It was a continent-wide breeding program under the orchestration of the kindly, efficient English viriculturist. The world would be better for his management.

He expected pushback. But naysayers of Galton's two proposals turned out to be fewer and farther between than he feared. The absence of negative reaction seemed to uncork something in Galton. And he began to churn out writings like this through the rest of the century: *English Men of Science: Their Nature and Nurture* (1874); "Theory of Heredity" a year later—wherein he again attacked cousin Darwin's pangenesis idea by making use of the ideas of agriculture; and *Inquiries into Human Faculty and its Development* (1883). In the last one, he finally unveiled the term for which we know him: "eugenics"—well-breeding, goodly parentage, some humans controlling the breeding of other humans.

Until his death, in 1910, Galton wrote hundreds of editorials, studies, papers, pamphlets, speeches, and books repeating the power of hard, inborn heredity. When Gregor Mendel's pea plant experiments reappeared in 1900, Galton and his disciples—for by the dawn of the twentieth century he had several—did not miss a beat. They had been promoting these ideas for years and were ready to unveil a comprehensive program. The flag they flew had a single word on it: not viriculture or stirpiculture, but "eugenics"—the unifying tree rooted in all other disciplines. Galton secured a small Eugenics Records Office on 88 Gower Street, London, in 1904. (Coincidentally, his cousin Darwin had lived on the same block six decades earlier.) When he handed over his small organization to Karl Pearson in 1907, it was renamed the Francis Galton Laboratory for National Eugenics and officially linked to University College London. The Eugenics Education Society launched in London in the same year.

> "All creatures would agree that it was better to be healthy than sick, vigorous than weak, well-fitted than ill-fitted for their part in life; in short, that it was better to be good rather than bad specimens of their kind, whatever that kind might be. So with men. . . . The aim of eugenics is to represent each class or sect by its best specimens."
>
> —Francis Galton, "Eugenics: Its Definition, Scope, and Aims"[14]

Yet, as H. G. Wells also identified at the Sociological Society of London in 1904, there was a critical problem with Galton's version of eugenics. Galton focused on wanting *more* of the good types to breed. But that was impractical: "Goodness" was just too vague, too hard to breed for. Humans bred animals for utility to humans; what was the correlate trait for other humans? Moreover, the "fit" couldn't even be convinced to follow the eugenics rules: For crying out loud, Galton himself left behind *no* children to improve the human stock! Therefore, Wells concluded, the only efficient solution was the one already percolating out of America. To improve the future, eugenicists must stop the bad from breeding at all.

> "Eugenics, which is really only a new word for the popular American term 'stirpiculture,' seems to me to be a term that is not without its misleading implications. . . . The implication is that the *best* reproduces and survives. . . . The way of nature has always been to slay the hindmost, and there is still no other way, unless we can prevent those who would become the hindmost being born. It is in the sterilization of failures, and not in the selection of successes for breeding, that the possibility of an improvement of the human stock lies."
>
> —H. G. Wells, comment to Francis Galton[15]

The Menace of the Feebleminded

Fear and irritation had long been growing among elites that the undeserving, the unredeemable, the racial minority, the foreign, the hereditarily poor, the inebriate, the mentally deficient, and the criminal would siphon resources and then leave a greater number of degenerate offspring behind. By the 1890s, these fears had grown to a fever pitch—perhaps, as Wells noted, most vocally in the US.

No factor contributed more to the fears of American physicians of the 1890s than the new appreciation for the complexities of heredity. "Feeblemindedness," though a poorly defined term from the early 1800s, expanded in usage by the end of the century. Physicians deemed the feebleminded as individuals capable of earning a living but, because of underlying instability, unable to manage themselves in an ordinary way. Hard to define, but you knew it when you saw it. Or at least experts did. But non-experts? The feebleminded could "pass" for normal. And these people were often asymptomatic *carriers* of degeneration, warned physicians.

Passing meant the feebleminded were free to operate in ordinary society, could freely marry, could have children. With enormous demographic shifts in the late nineteenth century—people moving from countryside to city, Ireland to England, Mediterranean to Northern Europe, Europe to America—the feebleminded could quietly pass through society without detection. And, with all that passing and mixing, chances increased for *both* parents to carry feeblemindedness. The resulting children, physicians believed, would end up much more severely impaired: the epileptics, idiots, imbeciles, alcoholics, and perhaps many of the hereditary criminals came from parents with milder traits, who were only carriers. Without going after the root cause—the feebleminded carriers themselves—no amount of treatment of the most mentally disabled would make much of a difference. In the long term, the pool would continue to generate more and more severely disabled people, more and more inebriates, more and more criminals and paupers littering the streets.

Could the state offer *permanent* custodial care for this burgeoning class of feebleminded? As both politicians and physicians complained, that seemed unlikely. If democratic representatives would not allocate enough public funding to incarcerate all the criminals, what hope was there that funding would be made available to deal with the mass of feebleminded individuals who could work, vote, have families, even run for office?

> "There are in the United States not less than 200,000 feeble-minded people; some good authorities, less conservative, say 300,000 . . . as many as 60,000 are women of child-bearing age. That home custody does not prevent these women from finding mates, either by marriage or otherwise, has been demonstrated times without number."
> —Lucia L. Jaquith, "The Menace of the Feeble-Minded"[16]

This tension is what irritated American advocates of Scientific Charity, or "New Philanthropy," as Albert O. Wright, president of the National Conference of Charities and Corrections, called it. New Philanthropy opposed funds of the wealthy being thrown at poor degenerates without measurable, tangible results. Improvements to asylums, prisons, schools, infrastructure—sure. But Scientific Charity "seeks for prevention as well as for cure," Wright insisted. And scientific experts declared the cause of pauperism and crime to be "essential," some "defect inside," not merely an effect of education or environment.[17] Therefore, to prevent an ever-larger strain on the wealthy philanthropic class, there could be only one acceptable long-term solution to manage the unfit: Prevent more of them. Philanthropists, ironically, were about to become some of the chief promotors of American eugenics. Their reasoning: "Unless we are prepared for the drastic measures of wholesale death or equally wholesale castration," Wright warned, "we must cut off defective heredity by the more expensive but more humane method of wholesale imprisonment."[18]

The First Eugenics Legislation

In the mid-1890s, taxpayers in the states of Indiana and Texas declared they would not financially support "wholesale imprisonment." So, lawmakers in both states proposed those "drastic measures": sterilization bills to eliminate the reproduction of degenerates. In other words, they opted for "wholesale castration." Those bills failed, though narrowly.

Then, in July 1895, the Connecticut legislature took a different angle and successfully passed the first eugenics bill in the history of a democratic state. Powerful state legislators officially committed to stop degeneration by keeping the undesirable from reproducing. Connecticut criminalized the marriage of, or sexual intercourse with, any "epileptic, imbecile, or feeble-minded." The state even made it illegal to assist in the marriage of "any pauper." The punishment? A stiff three years in the state penitentiary for the perpetrator, a fine of one thousand dollars (over twenty thousand dollars today), and a year in prison for each accomplice—including religious or civil officials who "countenance[d] any violation."[19] It was far beyond what Sir Francis Galton was able to accomplish over more than a decade of advocacy in Britain.

But that was only the start.

CHAPTER CCCXXV.

An Act concerning Crimes and Punishments.

Be it enacted by the Senate and House of Representatives in General Assembly convened:

SECTION 1. No man and woman, either of whom is epileptic, imbecile, or feeble-minded, shall intermarry, or live together as husband and wife, when the woman is under forty-five years of age. Any person violating or attempting to violate any of the provisions of this section shall be imprisoned in the state prison not less than three years. *Penalty for certain persons living as man and wife when woman is under forty-five years of age. Amended Chap. CCCI.*

SEC. 2. Any selectman or any other person who shall advise, aid, abet, cause, or assist in procuring, or countenance any violation of section one of this act, or the marriage of any pauper when the woman in such marriage is under forty-five years of age, shall be fined not less than one thousand dollars, or imprisoned not less than one year, or both. *Penalty for aiding or advising violation of preceding section.*

SEC. 3. Every man who shall carnally know any female under the age of forty-five years who is epileptic, imbecile, feeble-minded, or a pauper, shall be imprisoned in the state prison not less than three years. Every man who is epileptic who shall *Penalty for carnal knowledge when female is under forty-five years of age, in certain cases.*

Connecticut 1895 law criminalizing marriage between the unfit, the first eugenics law in the US

Two years later, on May 16, 1897, Dr. W. R. Edgar, a member of the Michigan state senate, introduced a bill to make mandatory, and without necessarily consulting with the patient or their caregivers, the surgical sterilization of criminals and degenerates. It was basically the sort of legislation Dr. Gideon Lincecum had drafted in Texas decades earlier. By the turn of the twentieth century, Dr. Edgar was not out on some lunatic fringe. He based the legislation on a broad survey he had conducted of almost every physician in asylums, jails, and prisons, plus hundreds of other physicians across North America. Of the nearly two hundred that responded to his survey, only *eight* expressed even a modicum of hesitation about involuntarily sterilizing the unfit. "We hold then, any plan or mode of treatment that will remove the cause should be tried," Dr. Edgar insisted.[20] Physicians had the responsibility to save civilization from degeneration before it was too late. With that great responsibility should come great power.

Dr. Edgar cited the criminal anthropology of "Lombrosi [*sic*]," plus the fears of degradation as introduced by Gobineau, Morel, and others, now reframed by the Zionist journalist and avid Lombroso follower Max Nordau in his tome *Entartung* ("Degeneration," 1892). Then Dr. Edgar reinforced his position by referring to castrations *already being done* around the US, with or without any law. American physicians had already prepared the soil for European ideas about degeneration and heredity to spring into eugenics.

Take the Kansas State Asylum for Idiotic and Imbecilic Youth, for instance. Cutting off defective lineages was already being practiced. Only a month after castrating one serial masturbator, the asylum's superintendent, Dr. Pilcher, castrated three more degenerate boys. Then, a month later, seven more—eleven in all, "with a marked improvement both mentally and physically." When Dr. Pilcher faced a public outcry, the Social Purity League of Topeka solicited testimonials in support. One of the boy's parents, overjoyed, wrote to the Kansas governor John W. Leedy, who passed on the message to the Michigan legislators considering Dr. Edgar's bill: "I believe every parent . . . would, after examining into the condition of those boys operated on and observing the improvement in their condition, request the same treatment extended to their boys."[21] Along with Kansas and Michigan, ten other states stood on the precipice of passing such legislation, reported Dr. Edgar.

"That all persons, male or female, who are now or who may hereafter become inmates of the Michigan Home for the Feeble Minded and Epileptic, shall be

> subjected to an examination, by a board of medical examiners to consist of three competent physicians, to be selected as hereinafter provided, with a view to determining the advisability of causing such persons to submit to an operation that causes asexualization."
>
> —"Asexualization of Criminals and Degenerates"[22]

Dr. Edgar's 1897 Michigan castration bill failed. Reportedly, the legislators feared that they themselves or their less intelligent constituents might become eligible for castration![23] Though Connecticut criminalized the reproduction of any "epileptic, imbecile, or feeble-minded" in 1895, Indiana didn't pass the first involuntary sterilization law until 1907. Still, Michigan signaled the future.

What was it that changed in the last decade of the nineteenth century that tipped controlling the breeding of the unfit from discussed and sporadic to more open and organized? In the US, where institutionalized eugenics first took root, factors included conservative reactions against immigration and civil rights gains for women and African Americans (however marginal), plus a growing awareness of ecological fragility. Americans could not continually expand the number of non-white mouths to feed without consequences for the rest. Resources *would* run out. Couple this with other widely held fears that "civilization" made modern white men "soft"—a trope repeated loudly by soon-to-be president and friend to eugenicists Theodore Roosevelt—and American state governments allowed enterprising physicians to take genital surgery to the next level.

PART 2

Making Eugenics a Science
(1899–1927)

CHAPTER 5

The Indiana Plan

A t the Indiana State Reformatory on the Ohio River, just across from Louisville, Kentucky, Harry Sharp became the first widely recognized eugenicist in the US. Interestingly, Sharp was not inspired by Francis Galton's eugenics propaganda. His conversion came via a fellow American. An 1899 article by Albert J. Ochsner, the nationally known and respected Chicago surgeon, reported two surgeries he had successfully completed in 1897 on two middle-aged men. They suffered from enlarged prostates and, in the first case, hemorrhoids. Ochsner endorsed European vasectomies instead of full castrations. In context, neither the surgeries nor the conditions of the men were all that noteworthy. Alfred Wood, a surgeon at the University of Pennsylvania, had listed over three hundred such surgeries in detail for the treatment of enlarged prostates that had been reported in France, Britain, and the US well before Ochsner's.[1] Had Ochsner added his patients to Wood's survey, neither the patients' conditions nor the surgeries themselves would have stuck out.[2]

But the reason Ochsner wrote his spring 1899 article—and the reason Harry Sharp read it that fall—had little to do with therapeutics. Ochsner revealed that he preferred vasectomies to castrations because they were *unobtrusive*. And because they were unobtrusive, he explained, they could be used to sterilize the unfit without the patients' really noticing. "Statistics show . . . that fully three-fourths of all crimes are committed by habitual criminals," Ochsner insisted. "If it were possible to eliminate all habitual criminals from the possibility of having children, there would soon be a very marked decrease in this class." Prisoners would barely notice their vasectomies, Ochsner assured readers. A revolution in crime reduction would follow, without resorting to castration. Then Ochsner went one better. He suggested physicians should also snip alcoholics, the mentally ill, sexual deviants (including homosexuals), and the generationally poor.[3] To a well-known Chicago physician like Ochsner, the unfit turned out to be quite a large group of people.

Six months after Ochsner published, Harry Sharp made incisions of his own. Nineteen-year-old "Clawson" from Missouri was the first to feel Sharp's knife. Why? According to Sharp, Clawson suffered from "masturbation." In that lingering moral panic of the Victorian era, Clawson came to Sharp in the reformatory clinic begging for a full castration to save his soul from the damnation of sexual pollution. Sharp was only too happy to oblige. He recalled Ochsner's April 1899 article and conducted a vasectomy instead of castration to stop Clawson's masturbating.[4] What's interesting is that according to Ochsner's April 1899 article that Sharp said inspired him, vasectomy *didn't* dent the sex drive in male patients—only full castration did that. So, it's curious that Sharp would offer it as a solution for Clawson's masturbation problem. Technicalities aside, Clawson's vasectomy on October 12, 1899, did eliminate his ability to reproduce. It took some weeks, and perhaps a second surgery (Sharp's memory was unclear on this point), but eventually the vasectomy "cured" Clawson. The masturbation slowed, his thinking cleared, school came easier.

Vasectomy had improved his entire "nervous system," Sharp reported. What's more, with the fever by which many religious converts burn, Clawson preached Sharp's surgery to his fellow inmates at the Indiana Reformatory. They came by the dozens to experience the freedom of Sharp's knife, he later claimed.[5]

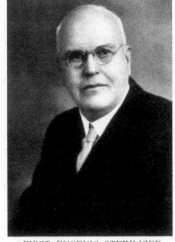

FIRST EUGENIC STERILIZER

Harry C. Sharp

Sharp cut—like Ochsner said he should, like other members of his profession already were doing. He claimed to vasectomize 176 men in their early twenties from 1899 to 1907, before the sterilization surgery became legal. No one with any real authority complained loudly enough, though, and Sharp remained silent about the procedure for those eight years.

If the number of degenerates was dangerously increasing, and vasectomy was so unobtrusive, why would Sharp not divulge? Fear of illegality might be one reason. For those who believe Harry Sharp was a eugenics innovator, much like those who believe Francis Galton created something new by coining the term "eugenics" in 1883, this explanation seems quite plausible.[6] However, if these surgeries to stem the tide of criminality and degeneration were becoming more common, as historical evidence suggests, and if the vasectomy was primarily therapeutic and only secondarily eugenic, Sharp may not have regarded his surgery on Clawson as all that groundbreaking.

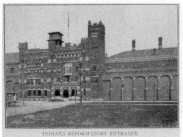
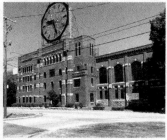

INDIANA REFORMATORY ENTRANCE

Indiana Reformatory where sterilizations took place, in the
early twentieth century and today

Indeed, it must only have seemed so once more organized
sterilization of the unfit fell under legal and scientific justifications, after the infamous Supreme Court decision *Buck v. Bell*
in 1927. This could be why no one bothered to interview Sharp
for thirty years, until 1937.

His interviewer at that time, William Kantor at Temple
University, in Philadelphia, clearly saw Sharp as a pioneer to
be emulated: "First legalized in 1907 by the Indiana Legislature, sterilization now is sanctioned in twenty-eight states
and in several foreign countries," crowed Kantor. Then, he
added—in a tone that can only be read today as ominous—
"notably Germany."[7] Of course, Kantor could not have known
that Third Reich physicians would soon use this American
knowledge to undertake "Aktion T-4," the sterilization and,
in many cases, extermination of hundreds of thousands of the
same sorts of "unfit" patients—the kind of patients Sharp and
others had begun sterilizing four decades earlier in the absence
of any distinct law passed by any legislature.

CHAPTER 6

The American Eugenics Triangle

The ideas about genetic determinism were already there. Physicians already cut. Sporadic laws already existed, and asylums already stood packed; prisons too. The feebleminded could be seen every day on American streets. Worries about crime by dark-skinned urban dwellers never really left the American psyche. But what made American eugenics a *movement* around the time of World War I turned out to be an organized web of actors.

A "Eugenics Triangle" of organizations hemmed together the northern half of the US and, from there, brought together much of the rest of the movement across the entire globe. On the eastern edge of that Triangle stood the powerful and well-funded Eugenic Records Office (ERO) at Cold Spring Harbor, New York. In the West was Paul Popenoe, Edwin Gosney, and David Starr Jordan's Human Betterment Foundation (HBF) based in Pasadena, California. John Harvey Kellogg's Race Betterment Society (RBS) in Battle Creek, Michigan, anchored the northern point of the Triangle. Not only did this Triangle of men, money, and institutions organize a relatively efficient eugenics propaganda operation (while ordinary physicians within the Triangle conducted the eugenic surgeries), it broadcast the message of eugenics far beyond the US—with disastrous consequences.

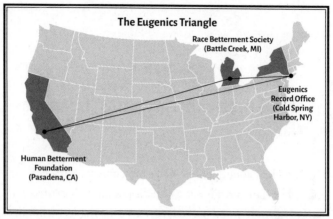

The Eugenics Triangle

Race Betterment Society
(Battle Creek, MI)

Eugenics
Record Office
(Cold Spring
Harbor, NY)

Human Betterment
Foundation
(Pasadena, CA)

The physicians, educators, and politicians within this network spread
the gospel of eugenics throughout New England, the mid-Atlantic,
Midwest, Great Plains, and up and down the West Coast. Texas
and the Southeast followed its own course.

East: The Eugenic Records Office

Of all the people involved, Charles B. Davenport was most
responsible for gathering geneticists and other scientists and
intellectuals into the eugenics movement. Davenport taught
biology at Harvard from 1892 to 1899 before leaving for a more
research-oriented post curating the zoological collection at the
University of Chicago's natural history museum. In 1902, he
contacted Karl Pearson, Francis Galton's eugenicist successor
at University College London and editor of *Biometrika*, the
preeminent quantitative evolution journal of the era. Through
Pearson, Davenport made connections to prominent biologists
throughout the UK and Europe. But when Pearson sharply
criticized Davenport's scientific conclusions in 1903, at the
height of the controversy between Pearson's Darwinian camp
and the new Mendelian genetics camp, Davenport sided with
the Mendelians.[1] Other American biologists began to view Davenport as a mathematically adept innovator, much like Galton

and Pearson, but easier to work with. That reputation launched him in 1904 from the University of Chicago's museum to head geneticist at the Station for Experimental Evolution in Cold Spring Harbor, New York, a preeminent experimental station used annually by hundreds of American biologists.

Tireless and opportunistic, Davenport traded on that position to expand his own network, then used it to lobby the vast wealth of the Carnegie and Rockefeller foundations, plus the E. H. Harriman railroad fortune. (John D. Rockefeller Jr., son of the oil tycoon, bankrolled the eastern half of the Eugenics Triangle through the first half of the twentieth century. Two of his sons, John III and David, played major roles in the international population control movement in the middle of the century.) Davenport was so successful that, for the first few decades of the twentieth century, he directed an endowment larger than all US university endowments for biological research *combined*.[2] He funneled a substantial portion of that money to his newly founded Eugenics Record Office (ERO); much of the rest went toward organizing international eugenics congresses to spread the word globally.

From New York's well-funded ERO, Davenport did what the British eugenics theorizers like Galton and Pearson could only dream of doing. He wrote, promoted, expanded, connected, and hired. He organized meeting after meeting,

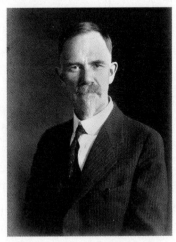

Charles Davenport

brought together geneticists and physicians and politicians and donors. He created multigenerational surveys, looking for traits that might be signs of degeneration. These surveys became the data set for his *Heredity in Relation to Eugenics* (1911), which argued yet again that "neuropathic taint" explained everything from alcoholism to poverty to racial inequality.[3] More than anyone, it was Davenport who smelted together the already existing practices of marriage planning and sterilization surgeries, Gobineau's racial fears, Galton's hard heredity, and the rest of the practices that had floated around medical and scientific culture for more than a half century. It was Davenport, in other words, who pulled together the scientific ideas and medical practices under one banner, christening all of it as "eugenics." And it was Davenport who dubbed the late Sir Francis Galton the "Father of Eugenics" and named Charles Darwin the inspiration for Galton, skipping over Victoria Woodhull, John Humphrey Noyes's Oneida Bible Communists, and any other claimants.

Like Galton, Davenport believed that inner biological essences, now called "genes," determined human traits, including intelligence, criminality, and mental illness. Because of these genes, certain groups of people were fated for particular roles in society. Aldous Huxley parodied Davenport's view in the novel *Brave New World* (1938), which depicts breeding farms for "Alphas"—society's leaders—and then those Betas, Deltas, and so on, down the ladder of human achievement. Huxley obviously drew from Davenport and from Plato's *Republic* to write his novel. But he had another, nearer source: his brother, Julian Huxley—a colleague of Davenport's—who promoted the eugenics movement in Britain through the first half of the century before becoming one of the major influencers in the United Nations after World War II.

Under Davenport's leadership, the ERO collected data on thousands of individuals and families, primarily through field studies, interviews, and surveys. They then used this data to compile a massive archive of genealogical and biological information on American families, the Eugenics Record Office Index. The ERO traced the genetics (they said) of criminality, alcoholism, feeblemindedness, and other deviant behavior in the hope of preventing those who could be carriers of these traits from reproducing. Standardized testing for intelligence, including IQ and SAT tests, though not developed by the ERO, were heavily promoted. Big data could help solve America's degeneration problem.

To call the ERO's influence "significant" is a massive understatement. Its work, as well as its messaging about deterministic, relatively simple biological essences and their impact on society shaped American medicine and jurisprudence for decades, particularly before World War II. Politicians, academics, and the media ceaselessly pushed these ERO-generated messages and used them to justify a range of policies that they believed improved the quality of the general population.

Of course, critics questioned the validity of the research conducted by the ERO, arguing that it was based on flawed assumptions and biased data. Others objected to eugenic sterilization. They noted that physicians driven by ERO publications targeted vulnerable populations, especially people with disabilities and those living in poverty. Nevertheless, the ERO only grew in strength until 1939, when support for the war effort, the priorities of FDR's New Deal, whispers of Nazi atrocities in the name of eugenics, and allegations of financial mismanagement channeled finances away.

Crucially, however, Davenport was not alone. The ERO could never have made the impact on American medicine and beyond without help. The Triangle made eugenics what it was.

Harry H. Laughlin

Davenport's right-hand man Harry H. Laughlin wielded

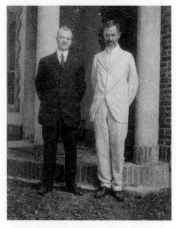

Harry Laughlin and Charles Davenport outside the new Eugenics Record Office building

the political lever of eugenics, translating the message of the Eugenics Triangle to state capitals and Washington power players. Davenport was a dedicated, Ivy League–trained scientist, a geneticist when that meant something cutting edge and a little intimidating. He compiled the data and managed the number crunchers from the ERO. He worked nonstop to boost the scientific credibility of eugenics and was successful in his own methodical way, proving to be the thumping heart of the eastern part of the Eugenics Triangle. If Davenport wove the web, Laughlin spidered its threads with a big midwestern grin and a firm handshake.

Laughlin had been a school principal, a superintendent, and an agriculture teacher (in that order). He excelled at glad-handing, backslapping, snapping his suspenders, and leaning forward affably while scratching his balding pate. Sure, he had studied cell biology at Princeton, and the full Windsor knot in his tie always stayed crisp. But he also knew regular-guy stuff. Farming, for instance. Horses, especially. He could talk thoroughbreds as well as work horses. And that amicable, open "aw, shucks" visage *sold* eugenics. No matter how full of flimflam, Laughlin could sway an audience, with every conversation a sales pitch—whether it be at county fairs, carnivals, or on Capitol Hill. If other eugenicists demanded his high-brow listeners live cleaner or know more science, all Laughlin demanded of his political friends was that they channel their power, not to manage their own constituents nor their paymasters, but to scrub the unwanted away.

And scrub they did. When Davenport appointed Laughlin managing director of the ERO in 1910, only a handful of states had eugenics laws on the books. At the time, only California pursued sterilization under the authority of their laws. Even Harry Sharp's Indiana had pulled back from organized, institutional surgeries (though physician-by-physician eugenics continued, however sporadic).[4] But Laughlin relentlessly pursued expanding sterilization. By early 1914, Nevada, New Jersey, Kansas, New York, Iowa, and North Dakota had joined the ranks of eugenics states. Michigan finally passed its own sterilization bill in 1913, almost two decades after Dr. W. R. Edgar's failed attempt. Laughlin forged valuable connections among physicians, politicians, social workers, YMCA directors, clergy, teachers, principals, leaders in the Scientific Charity Movement, statisticians, professors, and university presidents. The number of states adopting eugenics legislation skyrocketed.[5]

In the summer of 1920, members of the US Congress asked the ERO for help in bettering the race. Davenport sent Laughlin to Capitol Hill. As a result (which we'll see in a later chapter), the character of American immigration changed for the next four decades.

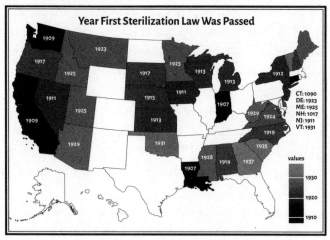

Year First Sterilization Law Was Passed

1909
1923
1917
1925
1925
1917
1913
1912
1911
1915
1911
1907
1909
1925
1929
1924
1913
1919
1931
1935
1929
1928
1919
1937
1907

CT: 1090
DE: 1923
ME: 1925
NH: 1017
NJ: 1911
VT: 1931

values
1930
1920
1910

Adoption of sterilization across the US prior to 1940

In his *Eugenical Sterilization in the United States* (1922), Laughlin drew up a "model eugenical sterilization law." Arguably, it would become the most tragically influential political creation of the entire interwar eugenics movement. Through it, Laughlin brought the American hope of curing societal degeneration by sterilizing weak, poor, and non-white people far outside the Eugenics Triangle as well as across the US.

Legal challenges to eugenic surgeries were already trickling in from various states, so Laughlin explicitly co-opted the language of cases and decisions to ensure that his model bill passed muster. First of all, no eugenics bill could be viewed as vindictive; no "cruel or unusual punishment" clause could apply: "Absolutely no punitive element," he stressed. Laughlin insisted that targets of eugenics bills could only be those inside and outside of prisons and mental institutions who "because of degenerate or defective hereditary qualities are potential parents of socially inadequate offspring."

Second, he called for a cadre of experts to oversee the "surgical operation upon or medical treatment of the reproductive organs . . . in consequence of which the power to procreate offspring is permanently nullified," with "due provision for safe, skillful and humane operation and treatment."[6] No politician, police officer, or prison warden kowtowing to a vindictive electorate or legal system could wield arbitrary surgical power. Sterilization had to be left up to the cool judgments of medical men, stressed Laughlin, and it would be best if it were an official state eugenicist.

Finally, Laughlin admitted that, while a case for eugenic sterilization could be brought against anyone suspected of harboring degenerate traits (yes, this meant an ordinary citizen could snitch on a neighbor, family member, or enemy), a judge and a six-person jury would have a say. Laughlin even included an appeal provision.

Confident, persuasive, friendly, measured, thorough, and well networked—Laughlin's demeanor and model law launched him into the national conversation. It's interesting to note that his big moment was not the institution of the Model Sterilization Act. That would take the work of others, like Dr. Albert Priddy (of *Buck v. Bell* fame; see chapter 8). Instead, Laughlin found himself embedded in anti-immigration work. Eugenics was tangled up with immigration from the beginning.

Midwest: The Race Betterment Society

Eccentric, charismatic, and indefatigable (though not the quack depicted in the novel or film *The Road to Wellville*), Dr. John Harvey Kellogg sat at the northern point of the Eugenics Triangle. From Battle Creek, Michigan, J. H. and his brother,

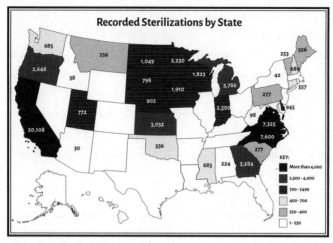

Recorded Sterilizations by State

685 · 256 · 1,049 · 2,230 · 253 · 326 · 2,648 · 38 · 1,823 · 689 · 42 · 798 · 3,786 · 557 · 1,910 · 277 · 902 · 2,500 · 945 · 772 · 98 · 3,032 · 7,325 · 20,108 · 7,600 · 30 · 556 · 277 · 683 · 224 · 3,284

KEY:
More than 4,000
2,500 - 4,000
700 - 2499
400 - 700
250 - 400
1 - 250

Number of officially recorded eugenic sterilizations in the US per state from 1907 to 1980: Note that untold numbers of sterilizations were never recorded due to poor recordkeeping, classification as other than "eugenic," or because eugenic sterilization was not legal in that state.[7]

Will Keith Kellogg, channeled their growing cornflakes cereal fortune into the Race Betterment Society (RBS). Will Keith eventually devoted his time entirely to the cereal business. But starting in 1877, J. H. ran the Battle Creek Sanitarium, a Seventh-Day Adventist retreat center turned "clean living" resort for the wealthy and troubled. The Sanitarium served as the beautiful and well-funded headquarters of the RBS. Guests received individualized attention from a team of devotees to Dr. Kellogg's methods and a regimen focused on a vegetarian diet (including Kellogg's Corn Flakes, meat being a gastronomic "death wish"), frequent enemas, and regular outdoor exercise. J. H. also expected his guests to abstain from sex, alcohol, caffeine, and tobacco, which he considered dissipations of the nervous system leading to degeneration.[8]

Clean living (which J. H. called "euthenics") did not preclude Kellogg from focusing on clean breeding, of course.

"Every teacher," proclaimed Kellogg, "every leader of human thought, every publisher, all professions, all serious-minded men and women should join in making known to every human being in every corner of the globe the fact that *the human race is dying*, and in seeking to discover and apply the remedies necessary for salvation from this dismal fate."[9] For Kellogg, demographic data pulled primarily from British records (since Americans hardly kept documentation that meticulous) demonstrated the slow demise of the white race. It was time to start breeding white humans as carefully as we breed dogs and chrysanthemums, urged Kellogg.

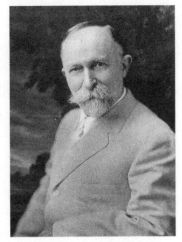

John Harvey Kellogg

But such a thing could not be done by force; he didn't like sterilization surgeries. Race betterment required incentives, not blades. Kellogg preferred sponsoring contests to discover the best, least degenerate, most biologically fit families. Indeed, "fitter family" and "better baby" contests would become as much a staple of the American eugenics movement as cornflakes was to our breakfast tables.[10] Kellogg's ultimate goal for these contests, however, wasn't to dole out awards alone, but to solicit data. Kellogg wanted a national registry of families, a pedigree chart that would allow for more intelligent breeding, which would be kept by the ERO.

Kellogg's push for a heredity registry became one of his two most important contributions to the eugenics movement in the early twentieth century. His other contribution was even more significant: national promotion. Kellogg hosted massive RBS conferences from his 1,200-room Battle Creek Sanitarium, advertised to the great and the good around the country. Henry Ford made use of it. So did Thomas Edison, J. C. Penney, Amelia Earhart, Sojourner Truth, and even the future presidents Warren G. Harding and William H. Taft. At the Sanitarium's RBS meetings, Kellogg connected the nation's most committed eugenicists, Davenport and Laughlin, for instance, to hundreds of the most culturally influential figures on the globe.

Not surprisingly, the First National Conference on Race Betterment held at Kellogg's Sanitarium in early January 1914 connected seventy high-profile speakers from across the Anglo-American eugenics movement. They engaged with topics ranging from the scourges of tobacco and masturbation to intransigent (because biological) poverty and "America's Oriental Problem." In his contribution to the conference, Charles Davenport echoed Kellogg's plea for data collection. But rather than contests or enemas or vegetarian living, eugenicists, Davenport insisted, wanted financial results. And they could deliver.

Eugenicists would help states shed enormous fiscal burdens of caring for the unfit through prevention. Science—Davenport's eugenics—would show the way. This message about money became one of the most enduring parts of the eugenics movement. And because of Kellogg's RBS, it filtered down to tax-averse captains of industry across the nation.

During his speech at Kellogg's 1914 conference, Davenport confirmed that surveys showed epileptics produced more epileptics; the insane made more insane children; criminals, more criminals: "from such localities where the degenerates are bred, go forth a stream of people who constitute certainly a large proportion of the paupers, beggars, the thieves, burglars and prostitutes who flock into our cities."[11] If somehow these worthless families could be cut off, every community—the whole globe really—would be well on its way toward greater health. No enemas necessary.

To be clear, by "race betterment" Kellogg believed in promoting, amplifying, and sharpening the fit. Kellogg, more so than Galton or Davenport, thought "nurture" still had an extensive role to play in improving the race. Historians have called this "positive" eugenics.

To the same congregation brought together by Kellogg, Davenport preached a lesson about halting the unwanted, the costly, the unworthy altogether. Davenport's message sounded more pragmatic—a way to cut costs, crime, and sexual deviancy that would have tickled the ears of Fords, Penneys, and Edisons in his audience. This has been called "negative" eugenics, and it drew energy from the promise that cutting nature would solve the problems that better nurturing could not. Kellogg's positive side required personal sacrifice, individual hard work, discipline, and intestinal fortitude (quite literally). Davenport's method, by contrast, followed in the long American tradition of those with power controlling the bodies of others with less power. It's no wonder "negative" eugenics won out.

West: The Human Betterment Foundation

In some ways, the western point of the American Eugenics Triangle mirrored the eastern. Dour and studious, Paul B. Popenoe gathered other serious-minded moralizers in

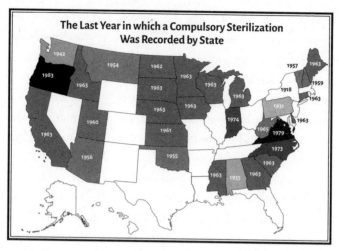

The Last Year in which a Compulsory Sterilization Was Recorded by State

The last year each US state recorded an official compulsory eugenic sterilization: Note that uncertain legal status in certain states meant that sterilizations could occur after these dates without being recorded.[12]

southern California around the Human Betterment Foundation (HBF). He founded it in the wake of Kellogg's Second National Conference on Race Betterment, in the summer of 1915. J. H. Kellogg had called again for a eugenics registry, and given that the conference took place at San Francisco's ostentatious Panama-Pacific Exposition and that the eugenicists had the largest booth in the place, Kellogg's message about marriage restrictions and healthy living spread to an even larger crowd than he had had in Michigan. Ezra S. Gosney, a citrus magnate inspired by the Second Conference, served as Popenoe's West Coast financial backer when the HBF was formalized at the end of the 1920s. By that point, Popenoe—very much like Davenport—had moved from agriculturalist to "geneticist." His *Journal of Heredity*, still in publication today, served as an effective blend of up-to-date science and eugenics advocacy.

Together, Popenoe and Gosney crafted *Sterilization for Human Betterment: A Summary of Results of 6,000 Operations in California, 1909–1929* (1929), the first major study of industrialized American eugenic sterilization surgeries. Unsurprisingly, the book showed how sterilizations of men and women proved to be both safe and effective. Competent medical men like Dr. F. O. Butler, head of the Sonoma County State Home in Santa Rosa, 50 miles (80 km) north of San Francisco, had confidently reported to Popenoe and Gosney that very few post-operative deaths or other undesirable outcomes occurred over the hundreds of sterilizations that he conducted at his facility beginning in 1919. (Butler personally sterilized or oversaw the sterilization of over 4,300 patients in 25 years, a sizable portion of all California sterilizations before World War II. His Sonoma asylum eventually became one of the leading eugenic sterilization facilities in the entire US.[13]) The book made an immediate splash. This promotion of eugenics proved so effective that German doctors began to seriously consider it, even before the early 1930s Fascist takeover.

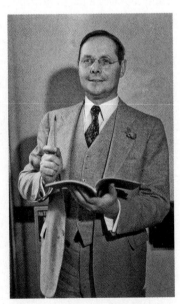

Paul B. Popenoe, who, with Ezra S. Gosney, helped lead the Human Betterment Foundation

Prominent West Coast individuals heeded Popenoe

and Gosney's eugenics call. Justin Miller, professor and dean at the University of Southern California School of Law, a future FDR appointee to the DC Circuit Federal Court of Appeals, and future president of the National Association of Radio and Television Broadcasters, played a starring role as founding member of the HBF. So did David Starr Jordan, a biologist and the founding president of Stanford University. Gosney convinced two dozen other prominent scientists, businessmen, journalists, and urban elites to spearhead the HBF. Once the California Institute of Technology (Caltech) got up and running in the 1920s, Gosney convinced prominent faculty and university donors to invest in and promote the HBF. Some, including the world-renowned physicist Robert Millikan, who won the 1923 Nobel Prize and then led Caltech for over two decades, became a major booster for eugenic sterilization. He joined the HBF board in 1937, by which time the Nazi promotion of eugenics ideas was well known the world over. When Gosney died in 1942, Millikan shepherded the funds of the HBF to Caltech. The Gosney Research Fund at Caltech would ever after support research into "the biological bases of human qualities."[14]

Without a doubt, the eastern side of the Eugenics Triangle had the most political impact in the first half of the century. But California took the lead in sterilizations. Between the wars, surgeons sterilized an average of 450 men and women annually. Laughlin tabulated over 14,000 by 1940—quadrupling Virginia, the next highest state.[15] And the heavy hitters of the HBF seemed to keep the press on the side of eugenics. The *San Francisco Examiner*'s stories about Popenoe, the HBF, and the eugenics movement in general were either decidedly favorable or used the eugenicists' own terms to describe social problems—society was degenerating because of defectives, hereditary criminals, the unfit, and the undeserving poor.[16] Not even open admiration for Hitler's "hopes of national regeneration" based on "the care of [Germany's] best racial elements" could sully Popenoe's reputation or the HBF's influence on the West Coast.[17]

The cultural impact of Popenoe's social engineering in the western half of the Eugenics Triangle lingered well beyond the ERO's influence. Dr. F. O. Butler's sterilization practices persisted well after the war in California asylums. And Popenoe transitioned to one of the foremost prophets of eugenic heteronormativity, as a nationally respected marriage counselor. Popularizing the eugenic family had been his goal all along, after all, and this new angle seemed like a smart way to do it.[18] Legitimizing only traditional sex and gender roles, his model of marriage counseling rapidly spread across the US in the 1940s and into the television age.[19]

Popenoe upheld traditional gender roles in *Modern Marriage: A Handbook* (1925) and *Problems of Human Reproduction* (1926). In those books, he extolled the virtues of Anglo-American middle-class heteronormative family life: dominant fathers and stay-at-home mothers who supplied the domestic needs of husband and children. From Popenoe's perspective, this eugenically sound arrangement not only made for greater happiness, it secured the preeminence of the white race.[20] Religious celibacy, Popenoe declared, was the true work of the devil because it ensured that the "inferior members of the race gave birth to the next generation . . . the race was perpetuated . . . only by the second-best." Only prostitution could be worse than celibacy as a generator of unfitness.[21]

Popenoe jumped into marriage counseling with both feet, opening his American Institute of Family Relations (AIFR) in Los Angeles as a first-of-its-kind counseling center, a "clearing house for problems of marriage and parenthood."[22] But he retained his eugenics connections: the American Eugenics Society funded Popenoe's AIFR. And he persisted in lobbying for eugenic sterilization, updating his *Sterilization for Human Betterment* (1929) with *Twenty-Eight Years of Sterilization in California* (1938), another unabashedly promotional piece. The 1938 book showed two trends: the first, that disproportionate numbers of non-whites were being sterilized, and second, that sterilizations were fast picking up in private practice rather than public institutions. We can't know whether these trends were effects of Popenoe's sampling or an actual move back toward unregulated, out-of-the-way surgeries, but the data are intriguing. Especially given what happened next.[23]

"Can This Marriage Be Saved?," one of the *Ladies' Home Journal*'s most popular series, was Popenoe's creation in the early 1950s. He wrote it as a trialogue: a wife's complaint, a husband's sometimes problematic response, and Popenoe's diagnosis (which almost always ended with the woman needing to adapt). The column continued even after the *Ladies' Home Journal* folded, in 2014. (In its present form as the pro–sex toy *More*, it would be unrecognizable to Popenoe.) In 1960, a best-selling collection of his essays appeared, refreshing his image as "Dr. Marriage"—despite the fact his "Dr." was a completely honorary one. (An English major, Popenoe had picked up genetics in college but dropped out before graduating.) He also frequently appeared as an advice-spouting guest on Art Linkletter's massively popular television show "House Party" through the 1950s. And in April 1957, he sat next to Miss Norway on Groucho Marx's television program "You Bet Your Life," dispensing his typical white professional class schtick.[24] By that point, Popenoe's dourness gave him the demeanor of a Very Serious Man that people needed to pay attention to, especially when discussing who should marry and have children.[25]

After the various cultural revolutions of the 1960s, Popenoe retooled again. Scrapping his earlier condemnations of religion as coddling the weak—but never shedding support for the eugenicists' heteronormative middle-class family—he began working with purportedly evangelical "pastoral psychotherapists." To a new generation, Popenoe passed on all those years of clean living and breeding in support of the white race to a new generation eager to cash in on the marriage advice industry.

For instance, in California in 1979, news appeared regarding a film series called *Focus on the Family*. Its creator, Dr. James C. Dobson, was a protégé of Popenoe's. The papers announced that Dobson's series was already "widely acclaimed by sociologists including Paul Popenoe, founder and president of the American Institute of Family Relations." Even after Popenoe's death and the collapse of mainstream eugenics, the sentiments of the Eugenics Triangle lived on through Dobson's conservative media.

Focus on Family Film Series Set

A film series titled "Focus on the Family" will start Sunday, January 27, at 6 p.m. at First Church of the Nazarene, Morrissey Boulevard at Gault Street, Santa Cruz.

For more information on the series call 423-3630. The series was filmed by Dr. James C. Dobson, teacher and psychologist, and has been widely acclaimed by sociologists including Paul Popenoe, founder and president of the American Institute of Family Relations.

Focus on the Family received a significant launch boost from the eugenicist Paul B. Popenoe.

CHAPTER 7

Studying the Worst of Us

The opposite image of Popenoe's ideal eugenic family appeared in over a dozen studies from the 1800s all the way through the 1920s. These families haunted every eugenicist, including Popenoe, for generations.

"In a small room I found an old blind woman, her son, his wife and two children, his sister with one child," began Reverend Oscar C. McCulloch, pastor of the socially active Plymouth Church in the growing town of Indianapolis. "There was no chair, table or stool, a little 'monkey stove,' but no fire; no plates, or kettles, or knife, fork or spoon. Such utter poverty horrified me." Reverend McCulloch was speaking at the National Conference of Charities and Corrections held in Cleveland, Ohio, in the summer of 1880. (Even the name of that organization gave away some of the conceptual changes; it had recently been the Conference of Boards of Public Charities—"corrections" didn't used to be a goal.) The good reverend instinctually knew what to do for the poor: "I soon had coal, provisions and clothing there." But McCulloch had also read the scientific literature. He knew about hereditary taint, how scientists traced currents of crime, poverty, alcoholism, and insanity through families. (Galton was still three years away from coining "eugenics," by the way.) Holding these suspicions in mind, McCulloch hunted for the blind woman's family in public records. There, McCulloch claimed he had stumbled upon the problem of unfit hereditary degenerates. He would pin a memorable name on them: the "Tribe of Ishmael."[1]

> "Here I found that I had touched one knot of a large family known as 'American Gypsies.' Three generations have been, and are, receiving public aid, numbering 125 persons; 65 percent were illegitimate; 57 percent of the children died before the age of five. . . . Since then I have found that family underrunning our society like devil-grass. In the diagram which I hold before you, the extent of it is traced to over 400 individuals. They are found on the street begging, at the houses soliciting cold victuals. Their names appear on the criminal records of the city court, the county jail, the house of refuge, the reformatory, the State prison and the county poor asylum."
>
> —Reverend Oscar C. McColloch, on his "Tribe of Ishmael"[2]

McCulloch's "Ishmaelites" were one of around twenty "families" studied from the 1870s to the 1940s by a loose collection of health care workers, government agencies, sociologists, anthropologists, eugenicists, and even pastors. Over the course of fifteen major studies and several smaller ones, authors gave those "families" memorable new names: Jukes, Kallikaks, Nams, "Smoky Pilgrims," and so on. Here is the full list of "families"; the study's central author and year are in parentheses.[3]

1. The Jukes (Dugdale, 1877)

2. The Tribe of Ishmael (McCulloch, 1888)

3. Smoky Pilgrims (Blackmar, 1897)

4. The Jukes-Edwards (Winship, 1900)

5. The Zeros (Gertrude Davenport, 1907)

6. The Kallikaks (Goddard, 1912)

7. The Hill Folk (Danielson and Charles Davenport, 1912)

8. The Nams (Estabrook and Charles Davenport, 1912)

9. The Pineys (Kite, 1913)

10. Sam Sixties (Kostir, 1916)

11. The Dacks (Finlayson, 1916)

12. The Jukes [revisited] (Estabrook, 1916)

13. The Hickories (Sessions, 1918)

14. The Coreys, the Yaks, and the Tams (Rogers and Merrill, 1919)

15. Mongrel Virginians (Estabrook and McDougle, 1926)

Importantly, many of those studied were *not* directly related (hence "families" should go in quotes) or had only a few distant relatives in common. Nevertheless, experts understood the biosocial lessons to be drawn. As Reverend

McCulloch put it, "The law of degeneration is as active as that of gravitation. No social student will question the existence of such a law of degeneration in society or has failed to see such degraded forms of life."[4] The assumptions of degeneration and determinism couldn't be questioned. McCulloch and his ilk simply rendered these "families" morality tales told in the language of statistics.

By the post–World War I era, the messaging rang out clearly in books, newspaper and magazine articles, sermons, and displays at eugenics congresses—isolate these groups, incarcerate many of them, withdraw funding, and restrict their breeding by any means possible.

Dugdale's Jukes

The original "family" study, however, emphasized different lessons. Twenty years before Reverend McCulloch's Ishmaelites, Richard L. Dugdale, a sickly but fervent advocate for more humane prisons, visited the jail in Ulster County, New York. His interviews revealed that six people, held there under four family names, were supposedly blood relatives. Court records then led Dugdale to believe that half of the forty or so male relatives of those six had also been convicted of a crime. Dugdale saw this as evidence, but *not* of degeneration and biological determinism. Instead, that a rough home environment, lack of meaningful work, and easy access to alcohol perpetuated criminality.

Dugdale *opposed* the messages about degeneration and biological determinism he heard from prison wardens and physicians. Trained in art, architecture, and new theories of social reform at The Cooper Union for the Advancement of Science and Art, in New York, Dugdale insisted that environment mattered at least as much as heredity.[5]

After a largely self-funded, multiyear study of 709 subjects in Ulster County, Dugdale uncovered a network of relationships among most of these individuals, whom he identified as members of forty-two *distinct* families. Yet in his reporting, he created a singular, fictional family at the heart of his book *The Jukes: A Study in Crime, Pauperism, Disease and Heredity* (1877). Historians have since reextracted the names and lineages of Sloughters, Ploughs, Millers, DuBoises, Clearwaters, Banks, Bushes, and so on, which were vacuumed up into Dugdale's study. But the damage was done. "Jukes" has served forever after as a symbol of societal degeneration despised by followers of Gobineau, Quêtelet, Lombroso, and their modern-day disciples.[6] They were, in the pejorative of the time, "white trash."

Yet, unlike arguments rooted in biological determinism, Dugdale blamed society itself for the poor state the Jukes found themselves locked into. Their degenerate state might be *persistent*, but not *permanent*. To alleviate their poverty and crime, New York State needed to invest *more* resources. Give

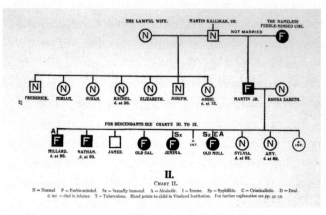

Kallikak "family tree," according to the eugenicist H. H. Goddard (1912): The "F"-designated individuals passed on "feeble-mindedness."

them shoes, clean water, healthy food, well-paid teachers, and not merely condemn them as hereditary degenerates.

It was, no doubt, partly because Dugdale blamed the poverty of the Jukes on the established social hierarchy that one of its members, Arthur Estabrook, revisited the Jukes study four decades later. Cynically, Estabrook, a full-throated supporter of Davenport and eugenics, inverted Dugdale's recommendations. Under Estabrook's 1915 rewrite of Dugdale's book—in which Estabrook included three times as many individuals as Dugdale—the Jukes became the model hereditary criminals draining elites like him of tax dollars.[7] According to Estabrook, the state's responsibility was not to help the Jukes out of poverty through the interventions of social workers, state agencies, and schools, but to limit their reproductive capabilities.

Rural Degeneration

Many of the mid-nineteenth-century worries about degeneration focused on cities for their supposed crime and disease. Phrases like "all rogues go to London" may have first gained popularity in the mid-nineteenth century. Yet, beginning with Dugdale's *Jukes*, the family studies singularly highlighted persistent degeneration in towns and rural areas. Ethnographic methods deployed by all authors of these family studies depended upon smaller, more stable family trees to make their point. Most of the fifteen major studies started with a living representative exhibiting undesirable behaviors or with an unsavory appearance. The author then traced lineages of these "families" back to white male "founders" using testimonies and local records in libraries and courthouses—a methodology impractical in large cities.

There were other practical considerations that made rural studies more attractive. Early eugenicists, Galton included, scooped up large amounts of data by conducting "contests" at mass public events. County fairs and agricultural shows proved especially fruitful for this method of personal data collection: Offer a prize for the "fittest" family or "best" baby, and hundreds of individuals will consent to give away a great deal of private information useful to eugenicists. Moreover, rural environments seemed safer for those sent to collect data. Though Dugdale and McCulloch conducted the work themselves, most of the later studies involved teams of research assistants or "field workers" sent out from the ERO on Long Island. These workers were often young, college-educated women. The moneyed interests funding the family studies preferred that these women steer clear of urban areas. (Note that John D. Rockefeller Jr. directly funded two of the most expensive studies himself.[8] The Rockefeller family would go on to be involved in eugenics and population control for the rest of the twentieth century.)

The multigenerational "family" stories almost always played out the same way. From that initial upstanding founder's relationships with questionable women issued increasingly shifty, uncouth, idle, dirty, mentally disturbed, and downwardly mobile descendants. The "families," no matter the name under which the eugenicists wrote about them, supplied farms and villages with prostitutes, thieves, drunks, bullies, beggars, the chronically ill, and other villains. Aside from their geographical locations and the particulars of their poverty, the "families" all carried the same inborn taint, a discrete genetic abnormality; it would never leave society, so long as the individuals bearing it were allowed to spawn their endless generations of degenerate children. The only true difference among these fifteen studies was the degree to which authors advocated intervention. Defunding or withdrawal of public support? Stricter laws? Larger asylums?

Mass incarceration? Marriage restrictions? Sterilization? Euthanasia?

CHAPTER 8

Legal Scaffolding for Eugenics

Workaday court cases and medical records reveal just how rapidly eugenics became a pervasive part of life in the US. Partly this shows the success of the Eugenics Triangle. But these cases also reveal that American physicians, especially those working in prisons and asylums, had quietly sterilized inmates for years without permission and without even mentioning "eugenics." Their targets were typically institutionalized criminals. But increasingly, physicians, prison wardens, and asylum superintendents pushed to apply eugenics to suspected deviants, including promiscuous women, the feebleminded, and homosexuals, outside the walls of any institution. What follows is only the visible tip of a eugenics iceberg.

State of Washington v. Feilen (1912)

The court found Peter Feilen guilty of raping a preteen child and sentenced him to life in prison. But the trial judge also sentenced Feilen to be sterilized by vasectomy. Feilen appealed, stating that sterilization violated the state's protection against cruel punishment. The Washington State Supreme Court disagreed. Not only was vasectomy a lighter sentence than the death penalty, to which others in his shoes had been sentenced, but it wasn't even as cruel as castration. The court cited some telling sources for its decision—not Davenport or Galton, but "the *Journal of the American Medical Association*," and "the Chicago Physicians' Club, the Southern District Medical Society, and the Chicago Society of Social Hygiene"—again emphasizing the degree to which punitive sterilization championed by physicians grew in parallel to, not necessarily in conjunction with, the proscriptions of the scientific eugenicists.[1]

> "On the theory that modern scientific investigation shows that idiocy, insanity, imbecility, and criminality are congenital and hereditary, the legislatures of California, Connecticut, Indiana, Iowa, New Jersey and perhaps other states, in the exercise of the police power, have enacted laws providing for the sterilization of idiots, insane, imbeciles, and habitual criminals. In the enforcement of these statutes, vasectomy seems to be a common operation.... We cannot hold that vasectomy is such a cruel punishment as cannot be inflicted upon appellant."
>
> —from *State of Washington v. Feilen*, 1912[2]

Davis v. Berry et al. (1914)

Judge Smith McPherson of the US District Court for the Southern District of Iowa disagreed with the *Washington v. Feilen* decision. Vasectomy might be a less invasive surgery than castration, but both were indeed cruel and unusual punishment and considered as such for centuries by English common law.

In 1913, the Iowa Parole Board instructed Austin F. Philpott, the Iowa Penitentiary physician, to vasectomize Adolph Davis. This procedure served as punishment for two separate felony convictions, though it also, according to Iowa's brand-new sterilization act, could be administered to those deemed feebleminded, alcoholics or "drug fiends," epileptics, syphilitics, or "sexual perverts." Judge McPherson found the penalty of sterilization cruel and unusual punishment. Physical suffering caused by the surgery, truly, may be minimal. Yet the social deterrent, which was exactly why physicians recommended castration in the nineteenth century, likewise made vasectomy cruel: "the humiliation, the degradation, the mental suffering are always present and known by all the public, and will follow him wheresoever he may go." Eugenicists classified vasectomy as the hallmark of modernity; but Judge McPherson concluded exactly the opposite: "This belongs to the Dark Ages."[3] Iowa appealed McPherson's ruling to the Supreme Court in 1914. But before SCOTUS weighed in, Iowa proactively weakened its law, and the Court remanded the case without passing judgment.

> "There is a difference between the operation of castration and vasectomy: castration being physically more severe than the other. But vasectomy in its results is much the coarser and more vulgar. . . . When Blackstone wrote his Commentaries he did not mention castration as one of the cruel punishments, quite likely for the reason that with the advance of civilization the operation was looked upon as too cruel, and was no longer performed. . . . The physical suffering may not be so great, but that is not the only test of cruel punishment; the humiliation . . . the mental suffering are always present and known by all the public."
> —from *Davis v. Berry et al.*, 1914[4]

But it's worth pausing on *Davis v. Berry* for another moment. McPherson predicated his emotional decision overturning Iowa's law on three grounds. First, on the respect for Davis's manhood; second, that sterilization could not be punishment for a crime; and, finally, that the individual to be sterilized must have due process before the law. As a response to *Davis v. Berry*, many states assembled more rigorous review boards of physicians and downplayed sterilization as a punitive surgery, thereby meeting the second and third of Judge McPherson's objections.

The first point is most telling, though. McPherson's empathy for Adolph Davis comes through loudly. But imagine that you could convince a judge or a parole board that the defendant isn't worthy of that level of compassion. Imagine that you could convince them that the accused was biologically, *categorically* different. This is exactly how the by-now-old degeneration narrative came to play such an outsized role in American eugenics, as we'll see in part 3.

Smith v. Wayne Probate Judge (1925)

Perhaps the first full-throated endorsement of sterilization for eugenics reasons rather than strictly punitive ones belongs to Michigan, the state that proposed the first American sterilization law, unsuccessfully, in 1897. By 1921, Indiana, just to the south, had declared its first eugenics law unconstitutional because, as in *Davis v. Berry*, it violated due process protections. The 1907 law championed by Harry C. Sharp had a good run, though, operating for more than a dozen years. Michigan judges distinguished their law from Indiana's by emphasizing the revenue-sapping degenerate wave. And that menace spurred states filled with pro-business, anti-taxation legislatures to pass new laws supporting sterilization not merely as an anti-crime remedy but as a means to contain government expenditures.

> "Science has demonstrated to a reasonable degree of certainty that feeble-mindedness is hereditary. This fact, now well known, with its alarming results, presents a social and economic problem of grave importance. . . . There are at least 20,000 recognized feebleminded persons in the State of Michigan. Eight times as many as can be segregated in State institutions. . . . That they are a serious menace to society no one will question."
>
> —from *Smith v. Wayne Probate Judge,* 1925[5]

Buck v. Bell, Superintendent of [Virginia] State Colony for Epileptics and Feeble Minded (1927)

Buck v. Bell stands as history's best known eugenics case. At first glance, the details appear straightforward. John and Alice Dobbs of Charlottesville, Virginia, attempted to institutionalize their foster child, seventeen-year-old Carrie Buck, at the State Colony for Epileptics and Feeble Minded, near Lynchburg, in January 1924. Teenaged Carrie, pregnant at the time, gave birth to Vivian Buck in March 1924. Carrie's mother, Emma Buck, also happened to be a resident at the State Colony. Alice Dobbs, who had used Carrie as domestic labor after caring for her since she was a small child, reported Carrie was feebleminded, though "moral delinquency" turned out to be a perfectly adequate charge, given that Carrie was pregnant.[6] (Everyone conveniently ignored Carrie's claim that she was

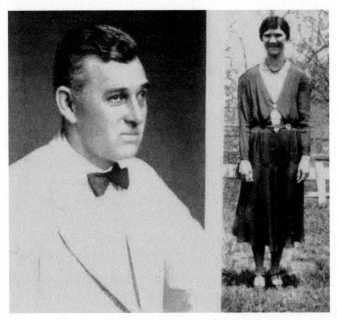

Buck v. Bell: Bell and Buck

assaulted and impregnated by a visiting Dobbs relative.) A small number of conservative physicians and attorneys headed by Dr. Albert Priddy, head of the Virginia Colony, pressured the state into a sterilization law based on Laughlin's "model sterilization law" explicitly to save the state money.

Carrie Buck proved an ideal candidate for testing the legality of Virginia's new eugenics law—designed specifically to pass Judge McPherson's objections in *Davis v. Berry et al.* a decade earlier. After stacking *both* the prosecution and the defense with attorneys and medical experts sympathetic to eugenics in general and the sterilization of feebleminded women more specifically, Priddy shepherded the case through the Virginia courts. Just before Priddy died in 1925, Virginia eugenicists handed off the case to a former West Virginia coal mine physician, a real company man, John Hendren Bell. Bell succeeded in pushing Priddy's case all the way through the US Supreme Court.

The court's nearly unanimous opinion, pronounced by Associate Justice Oliver Wendell Holmes Jr. in May 1927, amply summarized Bell's, Priddy's, and every other American eugenicists' feelings on the matter. But it also channeled almost one hundred years of Western fears about degeneration.

> "We have seen more than once that the public welfare may call upon the best citizens for their lives. It would be strange if it could not call upon those who already sap the strength of the State for these lesser sacrifices, often not felt to be such by those concerned, in order to prevent our being swamped with incompetence. It is better for all the world, if instead of waiting to execute degenerate offspring for crime, or to let them starve for their imbecility, society can prevent those who are manifestly unfit from continuing their kind."
>
> —Justice Oliver Wendell Holmes Jr., Supreme Court Majority opinion in *Buck v. Bell*, 1927[7]

Justice Holmes followed this reasoning with his infamous intonement: "Three generations of imbeciles [referring to Emma, Carrie, and infant Vivian Buck] are enough."

The court found eugenic sterilization, as proposed by Priddy and then Bell, did not violate the Fourteenth Amendment to the Constitution. According to the ruling, boards of experts would review each eugenics case. The surgeries were minor, certainly not cruel or unusual. And sterilization was not a punishment for a crime. Consequently, physicians sterilized Carrie Buck on October 19, 1927. Her sister, Dorris Buck, would be sterilized by J. H. Bell personally not long after.

What we sometimes miss in the retelling of the *Buck v. Bell* story is that the Supreme Court decision didn't end with that "imbeciles" quote. The justices also adjudicated the other portion of Priddy's original eugenics plans: to use sterilization to allow asylums to release inmates who could take care of themselves, work jobs, and so on, thereby opening beds to pull in more feebleminded from out of their own homes.

> "But, it is said, however it might be if this reasoning were applied generally, it fails when it is confined to the small number who are in the institutions named and is not applied to the multitudes outside. It is the usual last resort of constitutional arguments to point out shortcomings of this sort. . . . So far as the operations enable those who otherwise must be kept confined to be returned to the world, and thus open the asylum to others, the equality aimed at will be more nearly reached."
> —Justice Oliver Wendell Holmes Jr., Supreme Court Majority opinion in *Buck v. Bell*, 1927[8]

Cost cutting—the 1920s trend of shrinking the size of government rather than raising taxes to hire more staff or build more mental health facilities—was always part of the goal of Priddy's Virginia initiative that became *Buck v. Bell*. Indeed, Carrie Buck found herself "paroled" to another family to recuperate for a few weeks after her sterilization surgery, opening her space at the Colony to another patient.[9]

Scholars sometimes scold so-called progressive legislators, justices, and reformers for their blind spot about eugenics; take Holmes in the *Buck v. Bell* decision, for instance. But it's fairer to say the emotional drivers of this landmark case remained the same as those expressed by *conservatives* all the way back to Gobineau: fears of an immoral, crime-ridden society flooded by hereditary misfits that drained finances from the wealthy through government do-gooder policies warped by sentimental religiosity. While in *Davis v. Berry* (1914) Judge McPherson channeled empathetic disgust at the permanent dehumanization of sterilization, Justice Holmes and the seven other concurrent SCOTUS justices, including former President Taft, now the Chief Justice, did not share the same sentiment about the Bucks. Those of feebleminded ilk seemed not rise to the same level of humanhood.

Eugenics was never *just* about dealing with the mentally disabled. Bénédict Morel may have tried to disentangle race from degeneration worries all the way back in the mid-1800s.

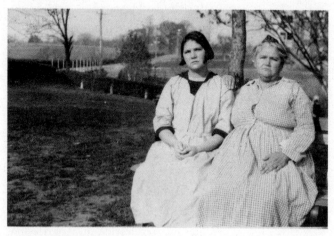

Carrie Buck with her mother, Emma, who was also institutionalized

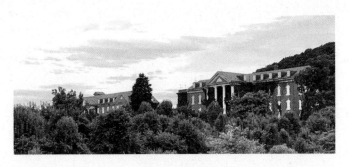

These derelict buildings of the Central Virginia Training Center
(originally the State Colony for Epileptics and Feeble Minded),
in Madison Heights, Virginia, were once a main site of eugenic
sterilization procedures.

But Gobineau's degeneration story never went away. "Racial
betterment" as preached by Kellogg and Popenoe, among
others, might simply mean eugenically selecting the best and
brightest, and not the poor or criminal, to carry on the next
generation. However, as we will see in part 3, racial betterment
often meant eliminating the non-white.

PART 3

Cleaning the Race

(1919–1945)

CHAPTER 9

Drowning the "Great Race"
Under a "Rising Tide of Color"

For a brief moment in the decade leading to World War I, eugenicists, especially in Britain, pretended racial prejudices could be disentangled from eugenics. But instead, old ideas of biological determinism and race intensified—all the way through World War II. Eugenics increasingly stretched beyond curing the individual family tree, to ranking, segregating, and purifying racial essences.

Observe, for example, the trajectory of Dr. Caleb Saleeby, a well-regarded obstetrician and a major influence on the eugenics movement in Britain. In 1904, he argued forcefully that the stress of child labor plus overcrowded cities led to behaviors detrimental to health, such as alcoholism and juvenile smoking. These, in turn, resulted in physical and mental wear and tear—we now use the term "weathering"—and, over long periods of time, lead to a degenerate population. None of the old, racist biological determinism could be found in Saleeby's straightforward treatise, *Physical Deterioration Being Mainly an Indictment Against the Cities of the Time* (1904). A mere three years later, in 1907, Saleeby, along with the elderly Sir Francis Galton, were early adherents of the first-of-its-kind Eugenics Education Society (EES) in London.

The deep fear of racial intermixing quickly twisted Dr. Saleeby. Gobineau's old complaint that Aryan interbreeding led to the downfall of civilization started to sneak through his writing almost as soon as he joined the EES. Over the course of several books—*Parenthood & Race Culture* (1909), *The Methods of Race-Regeneration* (1911), *Woman & Womanhood* (1911), and *The Progress of Eugenics* (1914)—Saleeby increasingly stressed that race trumped environment. To halt degeneration, whites must carefully manage their own reproduction so that the best in society would outnumber the worst. And, sadly, Saleeby proved to be one of the *gentlest* voices in the swelling eugenics movement.

Through the late nineteenth and early twentieth centuries, the old fears of degeneration mixed with existing racial prejudices in scientifically modern and, most important, very popular ways. Journalists, entertainers, high powered socialites, politicians, and captains of industry joined scientists and physicians in aggressively promoting eugenics. If the eugenics movement burned with a steady flame before, the works of these popularizers stoked it into a blaze. They also recentered the movement not merely on sick or dangerous individuals but on racial hierarchies.

Gobineau Rises Again Through Wagner's Followers

Gobineau Societies (*Gobineau-Vereinigung*), which incubated harsh views about defectives and Aryan racial purity, cropped up across German-speaking Europe after the German composer Richard Wagner traveled with an aging Joseph Arthur de Gobineau along the Mediterranean in the 1870s. Wagner fanned racial sparks lit by Gobineau in his monthly publication *Bayreuther Blätter* ("Bayreuth Pages"). On its pages in the 1930s, Wagner's supporters trumpeted the Nazi takeover of Germany as the purification of Aryanism and the arrest of racial degeneration.

Wagner's chief disciples, Houston Stewart Chamberlain, a British botanist turned Germanophile historian, and Christian von Ehrenfels, one of the founders of Gestalt psychology, loudly denounced interracial mixing using terms familiar to Gobineau. Their "races" were, on the one hand, those who carried the Aryan biological essence (soon said to be carried in "genes") and, on the other, those lesser whites from outside German-speaking lands who didn't have the proper essence (or genes). By mixing with these lesser whites, Aryans were degenerating. In this weakened state, whites would be outbred by the "Yellow Peril," the polygamous and fecund race of East Asia. Japan's unexpected victory in Manchuria in 1905 against the massive Russian Empire only confirmed their suspicions.

But a biological takeover by East Asian populations, however terrifying, loomed many decades to centuries in the future. In the meantime, Chamberlain, Ehrenfels, and other Gobineau-Wagner followers targeted a much closer threat to their white reproductive supremacy.

In April 1885 in London, the *Photographic News* published several composite images built from more than a dozen photographs of Jewish schoolboys. The photographs were taken by Joseph Jacobs, a local anthropology student and Hebrew scholar. His London-based instructor, none other than Sir Francis Galton, superimposed Jacobs's images on each other to create the smooth composite images. (Our era's AI-driven photography apps in a sense re-create Galton's Victorian-era technique.) These scientific images, Jacobs hoped, would combat the tide of growing antisemitism in Britain, because they showed that the "Jewish type" looked ordinary, normal, healthy, clean, and nonthreatening. Moreover, Jacobs, who established multiple Jewish mutual aid societies in the UK and the US, and published the landmark *Jewish Encyclopaedia*, saw in Galton's composites evidence of racial purity that, for the sake of the Jewish race, should be preserved. Jews, concluded Jacobs with Galton's technical support, stood *biologically*—as well as culturally and religiously—apart.

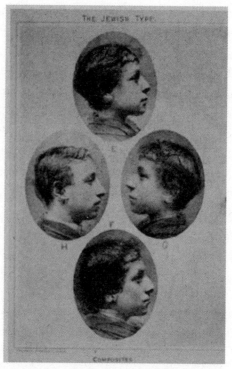

Galton's composites for Jacobs's paper "On the Racial Characteristics of Modern Jews," first published in the Photographic News (1885), were a technologically sophisticated attack on British antisemitism. Ironically, German, English, and American racists found "the Jewish type" helpful to their cause.

> "If these Jewish lads, selected almost at random, and with parents from opposite parts of Europe, yield so markedly individual a type, it can only be because there actually exists a definite and well-defined organic type of modern Jews. Photographic science thus seems to confirm the conclusion I have drawn from history, that there has been scarcely any admixture of alien blood amongst the Jews since their dispersion."
>
> —Joseph Jacobs[1]

But this is precisely what Chamberlain and Ehrenfels, among the other Wagner-infatuated promotors of Gobineau's degeneration myth, insisted as well. They ironically seized on Jacobs's photographs to undercut his anti-antisemitic hopes. Chamberlain and the Gobineau-Wagnerites promoted what accounted to salvation through the purification of Aryan whiteness and the concerted suppression of non-whites—especially the Jewish race. This race had now been "proven" to be biologically distinct by both history and the scientific photography of Jacobs and Galton. But the Gobineau-Wagnerites expressed displeasure that German and Scandinavian countries showed so little initiative in racial purification. The UK was even worse—an actual biological Jew, Prime Minister Benjamin Disraeli, ran the British government for years! In other words, antisemitism blended seamlessly into eugenics solutions.

> "All is race; there is no other truth. . . . The decay of a race is an inevitable necessity, unless it lives in deserts and never mixes its blood."
>
> —Prime Minister Benjamin Disraeli[2]

Chamberlain and Ehrenfels found a model for how to handle the Jewish "problem" across the Atlantic. The US had already enacted racial purity laws: the Chinese Exclusion Act of 1882, for instance. Americans also seemed to appreciate the evolutionary stakes of race war. President Teddy Roosevelt, among others, derided "soft" American whites. Like Chamberlain, Ehrenfels, and their racist colleagues, Roosevelt believed only the strenuous, manly life tied to the land on the "western frontier" could scrub the Aryan race clean, especially in preparation for its Darwinian struggle for supremacy against other races.

The American Influence

Meanwhile, two influential American authors in particular, Madison Grant and Lothrop Stoddard, used their personal platforms in New York City at the beginning of World War I to amplify racial fears in books read all over the world. Their writings were so successful that the embers of scientific racism tied to eugenics caught fire all over the globe, especially in Central Europe.

Madison Grant (1865–1937)

In the 1910s, Madison Grant, a Manhattan old-money socialite, and his close friend Henry Fairfield Osborn, the president for twenty-five years of the American Museum of Natural History, published a one-two punch of books repopularizing Gobineau's worries of racial degeneration for American audiences. Osborn, who was a nephew of J. P. Morgan and a member of Teddy Roosevelt's Boone and Crockett Club, published the five-hundred-page *Men of the Old Stone Age* in 1915. The tome became a standard part of high school and university curricula in the US for decades. In it, Osborn mirrored an equally racist if more sophisticated version of Gobineau: Cro-Magnons, a blue-eyed, intelligent, and muscular Paleolithic ur-race, were tragically displaced by fast-breeding, darker, lesser races in the "alpine" and the "Mediterranean" portions of Europe. Osborn's account of degenerative human history appeared at international eugenics exhibits. (His Gobineau-esque account has incredible staying power: I witnessed scientific illustrations essentially identical to Osborn's in my child's classroom nearly one hundred years after Osborn created them!)

Madison Grant's adaptation of Gobineau's theories had more sinister consequences. Adolf Hitler called a German translation of Grant's *Passing of the Great Race* (1916) his "Bible." In the Nuremberg "Doctors' Trial" after the Holocaust, Hitler's personal physician, Karl Brandt, held up Grant's book as defense of his heinous actions, including human experimentation and euthanasia. *You Americans did this first,* he charged.

Like Osborn's paleontology text, Grant's *Passing of the Great Race* repeated the old canard that a virtuous Aryan or "Nordic" race had long been forced to accommodate darker and dirtier "alpine" and "Mediterranean" races. Grant, who ran the New York Zoological Society and launched the American environmental movement,

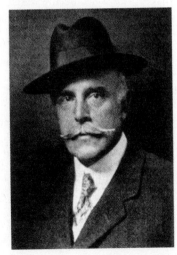

Madison Grant

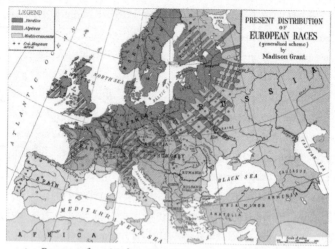

Race map from Madison Grant's Passing of the Great Race

firmly believed that every lasting technical, artistic, and intellectual achievement ascribed to Western society, including science itself, sprang from this "great race" of Nordics. But that greatness had been watered down through interbreeding, just as Gobineau had warned. Even pure-seeming Nordics exhibited hereditary mental illnesses and other degenerative symptoms common in lesser groups—a kind of "race suicide." The few pure Nordic groups left occupied only those pockets of northern and western Europe that spoke German-derived languages, including English. Some of their preeminent representatives transplanted themselves to North America, where they became, in Grant's telling, the mightiest families of the US and Canada.

Though he was neither a scientist nor an institutional leader in the Eugenics Triangle, Grant's open racism decisively bent the official eugenics movement during his tenure as editor of *The Eugenical News*, a central journal in the movement. In the 1910s, before Grant's involvement, the journal focused on degenerate *individuals*; during Grant's tenure as editor in the 1920s, the journal increasingly published stories decrying race mixing and the inferiority of non-white *groups*.[3]

Grant's *Passing of the Great Race* became a white supremacist manifesto every bit as influential as Gobineau's work eighty years earlier—perhaps even greater. Because, unlike Gobineau, Grant self-consciously touted his dispassionate method crafted as precisely as a twentieth-century treatise in physics or biology. He began with a hypothesis, that "race lies today at the base of all the phenomena of modern society, just as it has done throughout the unrecorded eons of the past." Then Grant "tested" that hypothesis with historical data. For instance, when did Alexander the Great's empire fall? The answer: when "pure Macedonian" blood mixed with "Asiatic" blood. Why did Roman civilization have such interclass conflict? Because Roman rulers descended from the Aryans (i.e., "Nordics"), while the plebeians were of the "Mediterranean race." Why did Spain lose its grip on a hemisphere-spanning empire? Because superior Nordic-Celtic blood mixed with Mediterranean blood in the Iberian and even "lower" races in the New World.[4] As much as Gobineau bemoaned the degeneration of France, and Wagner wept for Germany, Grant warned that Nordics in the UK and the US—a whole species, *Homo europaeus*, he insisted—were on the verge of being replaced by darker races. After hundreds of pages of "data," Grant insisted that the scientific hypothesis of racial degeneration had been scientifically verified.

Theodore Lothrop Stoddard (1883–1950)

The New York City journalist T. Lothrop Stoddard read *Passing of the Great Race*, and it changed his life. With a doctorate from Harvard, and a KKK robe in his closet, Stoddard went beyond Grant to investigate the incursions of non-white races on the world stage. Stoddard also used Darwinian rhetoric more seriously than Grant. In his two popular books that adopted the pretense of scientific objectivity, *The Rising Tide of Color: The Threat Against White World Supremacy* (1920) and *The Revolt Against Civilization: The Menace of the Under-Man* (1922), Stoddard aimed to frighten his Anglo-Saxon readers. Nonwhite folks were outbreeding whites all around the world. Darwinism, Stoddard reminded his readers, is a law of reproduction. And if a population loses the battle of reproduction, there is no amount of education, sanitation, or social engineering that can save it. Political consequences of this biological reversal could already be seen. The Bolshevik Revolution in Russia demonstrated what happened when a Jewish conspiracy of the clever and the complacent upended proper white rule. What would happen if those Jews and other Bolsheviks organized the lesser "races of

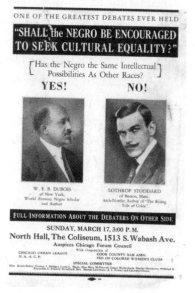

T. Lothrop Stoddard (right) debated the formidable scholar W. E. B. Du Bois (left) in this NAACP-sponsored event in Chicago (March 1929).

color" against whites? Maybe populations in the Middle East and Africa would revolt against European hegemony. Maybe the Philippines would throw off the US yoke. Maybe India would purge the British. Maybe one day a white man would be exhibited in a zoo—the way that the Congolese man Ota Benga had been displayed in Grant's New York Zoological Park. Imagine the shame if whites didn't take firm control of global breeding!

While it's easy enough to dismiss some of Stoddard's views as run-of-the-mill racist fare, he popularized more scientific-seeming genetic determinism. Geneticists could locate essences of intellectual inferiority, he believed, essences that were hardcoded into different races. Some versions of whiteness and some entire non-white races, as Grant pointed out, carried so much of this genetically inferior genetic essence that it made them permanently degenerated—the "under-men," Stoddard dubbed them.

And if this genetic determination weren't bad enough, warned Stoddard, Marxists, socialists, communists, and their muddle-headed do-gooder comrades wanted to overthrow those aristocratic, capitalistic, and colonials who kept the "under-men" down. The real threat of communism, as demonstrated by Bolshevism, wasn't merely a political or economic one. Communism, according to Stoddard, meant global biological degeneration and genetic race mixing. Crafty Jews, softhearted Christians, and anti-government anarchists would displace Nordics from the world stage using prolific Italians, Arabs, Asians, and Africans. Without swift and severe intervention, Darwinian evolution practically demanded this result.

Thankfully, Stoddard reassured his readers, eugenics undercut any version of Marxism, anarchism, or soft religious sentiment. Those "environmental" philosophies posit that social improvement comes from *outside*: by changing structures of power or educating individuals. "Eugenics," crowed Stoddard, "plans to improve the race *from within*, by determining *which* existing individuals shall, and shall not, produce succeeding generations." According to Stoddard, this view would be so much more effective and economical in the long run. "Improvements due to environment alone require

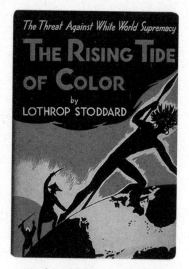

The first of Stoddard's influential books, *The Rising Tide of Color*, influenced President Warren G. Harding, energized Nazis, and became a talking point in *The Great Gatsby*.

a constant expenditure of energy to maintain," Stoddard highlighted. What's more, charity made maintaining social improvements worse by allowing the "incompetent" to genetically weigh the system down.[5]

National and International Impact

Madison Grant already stood at the top of New York's social ladder. But Lothrop Stoddard was launched into public prominence with his books. *The New York Times* glowingly reviewed *The Rising Tide of Color* over nearly a full page: "The East will see the West to bed," the *Times* reviewer fretted, "with Bolshevism menacing us on the one hand and race extinction through warfare on the other."[6] Even the US president, Warren

G. Harding, mentioned Stoddard's work. Eugenics tied to race science, President Harding intimated in his 1921 semicentennial speech in Birmingham, Alabama, would guide US policy.

> "Whoever will take the time to read and ponder Mr. Lothrop Stoddard's book on *The Rising Tide of Color* . . . must realize that our race problem here in the United States is only a phase of a race issue that the whole world confronts. . . .
>
> "Men of both races may well stand uncompromisingly against every suggestion of social equality. Indeed, it would be helpful to have that word 'equality' eliminated from this consideration; to have it accepted on both sides that this is not a question of social equality, but a question of recognizing a fundamental, eternal, and inescapable difference."
>
> —President Warren G. Harding[7]

To take another measure of the influence of these two pro-eugenics racists, look at American pop culture in the era. The very first issue of *Time* magazine, March 3, 1923, featured a full-page ad for Stoddard's works. Then, two years later, F. Scott Fitzgerald's classic novel *The Great Gatsby* (1925) immortalized them both. Tom Buchanan, the athletic, white, all-American rival to Jay Gatsby, blurts out, "Civilization's going to pieces. I've gotten to be a terrible pessimist about things," echoing generations of fears about degeneration. But then Tom offers the new scientific diagnosis: "Have you read 'The Rise of the Colored Empires' by this man Goddard?" (Goddard being a portmanteau of Grant and Stoddard). "These books are all scientific. . . . [It's] up to us, who are the dominant race, to watch out or these other races will have control of things."[8] Though Fitzgerald clearly didn't support the view—the rest of *Gatsby* makes that clear—Tom's lines showed that Fitzgerald grasped the popular reach of Grant and Stoddard.

These books made such an international impression that the Nazi regime rolled out the red carpet for Stoddard in 1940. During the first few months of the war, they invited him, alongside a few dozen Anglo journalists, to step behind the curtain of the Third Reich. (Madison Grant, the author of Hitler's "Bible," had died a few years earlier, or he would have toured Nazi Europe as well.) Through a network of Nazi race scientists (more on them later), Stoddard spent a day seated alongside the three justices on Germany's Eugenic Supreme Court in Berlin—built according to Laughlin's specifications in his Model Sterilization Act. The German high court failed to recommend sterilization in the cases brought before them that day. While Stoddard admired German efficiency, he judged the justices "too conservative."

Still, the more Stoddard traversed Germany in 1940, the more impressed he became. Clean streets; clean people, as he saw it. And, as he shook hands with the masters of Nazi propaganda, including having an audience with Hitler himself, he sensed mutual admiration. Here he stood in the middle of a whole nation successfully eliminating crime, poverty, filth, and inefficiency not merely by throwing social services and education at the problem, and certainly not by extending greater power or resources to the non-white "under-men," but by surgically extricating those who carried the biological essences of degeneracy from the gene pool. Certainly, he witnessed some unsettling sites: the inhabitants of shabby Jewish ghettos shot conspicuously terrified glances at the Nazi custodians accompanying Stoddard and the other journalists. But, overall, Stoddard thought, the Third Reich was rapidly crafting the eugenics standard for modern societies. He couldn't help but smile underneath his pencil-thin mustache.

CHAPTER 10

A Global Eugenics Network

Physicians and scientists who advocated eugenics had some decisions to make in 1918, at the end of World War I. With at least fifteen million soldiers and civilians dead across Europe, should German and British eugenicists put nationalism aside to rally around their mutual cause of stopping racial degeneration?[1] Immediately after the war, some of the most influential British and French eugenicists held on to their animosities. Scion of London's eugenics movement, Major Leonard Darwin, "sapper" (Royal Engineer) and distinguished son of Charles, stood fiercely opposed to German inclusion, openly arguing against even considering extending invitations to German eugenicists for the Second International Congress of Eugenics in 1921. That's why, when the Congress did take place, it was in New York City at the American Museum of Natural History. Major Darwin got his wish: no German eugenicists.

It may not have seemed so at the time, but this was the moment when any pretentions that eugenics was *British* went out the window. Major Darwin's objections did not deter the Americans at the Eugenics Records Office from orienting the entire movement. With his eye steadily focused on the greater good of racial purity, Davenport, leader of the ERO, hounded Major Darwin all through the Congress about the Germans and about financial support and about promoting the movement in the flashy American sort of way rather than the quieter English sort of way. In the end, Davenport triumphed. Germans would be readmitted to the movement in the later 1920s. More than that, the US became the hub of a global eugenics network that would last until the Great Depression.

Showing the Eugenics Narrative: The Second International Congress, New York, 1921

The single most complete expression of the eugenics story marketed by that American Eugenics Triangle and seeping into every national expression of eugenics appeared in the exhibition at the Second International Congress of Eugenics in the Forestry Hall (renamed "Darwin Hall" by the eugenicists) of the American Museum of Natural History (AMNH) in New York City in September 1921. Two decades after Harry Sharp's vigilante vasectomies, eugenics had bloomed into an international movement. The AMNH exhibition is how the eugenics movement wanted itself to be seen. Through the

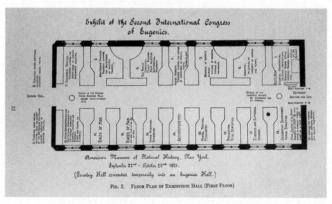

Second International Congress of Eugenics floor plan
(American Museum of Natural History, New York)

1920s, international eugenics looked increasingly like American race-centered "eliminate the worst" eugenics, rather than Galton's English "encourage the best" eugenics.

Imagine we were in the hall at the Second International Congress of Eugenics. If we followed the counterclockwise path of museumgoers, we could "read" the story of international eugenics in the early 1920s.

Early in our counterclockwise stroll, we encounter stories of hereditary greatness. These studies of "aristogenic" families represented the exact opposite of the "family studies" of the Jukes, the Tribe of Ishmael, and so on. At the top of the list stood genealogies of the *Mayflower* pilgrims and other prominent families in American history. Tragically, according to eugenicists, the lineages of these great American paragons might soon go extinct, threatened by indiscriminate breeding with lesser races. Among other goals of the Second International Congress, eugenicists indicated they fervently hoped to make America great again.

To do that, citizens needed more scientific knowledge. They would start by understanding how traits pass down in plants and animals. So, continuing around the AMNH exhibit, visitors encountered explanations of zoological and botanical genetics. One panel mentioned how negative mutations of genes could submarine as "recessives," carried for generations unless "pure line" breeding stopped the "admixture." If you could get the audience to accept this more neutral proposition, then you could move on to humans.

Booth 7 displayed the evil opposite of the *Mayflower* lineages: genealogical case studies of families harboring those underground defective "recessive" traits. "Cacogenic," the eugenicists labeled them. Reverend McCulloch's Tribe of

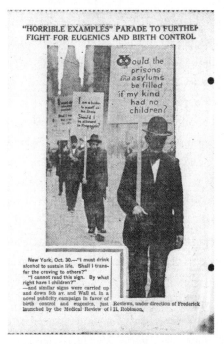

A New York eugenics awareness-raising campaign by F. H. Robinson

Ishmael, Arthur Estabrook's more biologically deterministic revision of the Jukes, replacing Dugdale's softer original. Then, Henry Goddard's Kallikaks, and the Dacks, Nams, and so on—each family a paragon of degeneracy, parasites on the public.[2]

Across from the "cacogenic" families stood Osborn's "Races of Man" exhibit. The paleontologist deployed skulls and archaeological artifacts to tell the story of European Cro-Magnon's dominance over the more apish Neanderthals. Unsurprisingly, the cacogenic families exhibit nearby displayed similarly apish "degenerate qualities" in contemporary faces. In the anthropometry exhibit, the same qualities indicated one's racial propensities and determined behaviors—the tendency to be a criminal, for example. This exhibit deftly blended eugenics with what is traditionally labeled "race science" in biological anthropology—a trend that would continue for decades afterwards in university anthropology programs from Harvard to Stanford.

The next booths contained exhibits on the dangers of immigration, the promise of intelligence testing (the Stanford-Binet Intelligence Scale predominated by the end of World War I), anthropometry—measuring skulls and bodies of the living, and the need for greater health hygiene, which included formal courses on hygiene in schools (called "health class").

Anchoring the entrance and exit points to the hall at the opposite ends, visitors passed two prominent statues. One was a composite sculpture of the "average young American male." Charles Davenport had commissioned his daughter, Jane Davenport Harris, to build a two-foot-high plaster statue of white veterans of the recent World War. Her reference points had been physical measurements collected from almost 100,000 veterans after their decommission in 1919, plus the results of the Alpha (words and pictures) and Beta (pictures only) intelligence tests administered to 1.7 million army recruits from 1917 to 1919. The results of that data collection turned out to be surprisingly unflattering. American fighting men were even weaker, sicker, shorter, and less intelligent than prewar reports suspected. The eugenicists' long-prophesied degeneration—which Jane Davenport Harris's statue portrayed—had already set in.

At the other end of the hall was another composite statue, this one created from the "50 strongest men of Harvard."[3] Unlike the "average" man it mirrored, this composite gleamed as the apex: unsullied white masculinity, possessors of eugenically pure, athletic, intelligent genes.

I'm taking you on this imagined lap around the exhibits for the Second International Congress of Eugenics to show that, in the wake of World War I, concepts that had floated around for a century now hardened into a unified narrative. One that was built on evidence from so many fields, so much common sense, so much artistic expression and common cultural clichés, and one that was layered

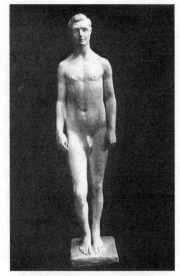

The Average American Male, according to statistics compiled through World War I tests and eugenicists at the Second International Congress of Eugenics

with so many statistics and hard genetic data. In this hall, now named in honor of Charles Darwin, through roughly twenty little rooms arranged like frames in a movie, scientists, physicians, policymakers, educational officials, and hundreds of volunteers wove together a eugenics master narrative.

The Eugenics Master Narrative

The narrative echoed Grant and Stoddard and on and on, back at least to Gobineau, though the organizers primarily hooked on to Galton and Darwin. Here's the core narrative as eugenicists and their followers intended us to understand it.

Some people, because of the deep propensities of their race and/or the maladaptive traits they carry within, are determined to be inferior to others. It's *not* the legacy of slavery or discrimination or malnutrition or overwork or wealth disparities. And it's not the fault of capitalistic colonizers from America and Europe. It's not even the fault of the environment. *It is biology.* Given the long history of humankind, ranking and inequality—plus the seeming injustice and oppression that follows from it—is *natural*, simply a part of our species' genetic story. There is little that education or social planning can do for those lesser individuals or even whole races.

Yet there are also more subtle negative traits that float through all races, even the white race, traits we can sift out. In other words, we can redeem whites and hold back the tide of degeneration over several generations if we can locate those negative traits. That way, whites can remain on top in the Darwinian war of the races. Scientists have developed ways—by experts in psychology administering objective intelligence tests, for instance—of detecting defects, of pulling out those who would otherwise "pass."

Those with mental or physical defects should not be permitted to leave those defective traits to children. Even mildly

	Families of the parents of college students	Dysgenic families in which the mothers are 45 years or older
Average number of births	3.28	7.91
Average number of children not living	0.44	1.74
Average number of children living	2.83	6.17
Birth interval	7.3 yrs.	3.1 yrs.
Percentage of survivals	80.3	77.9

Statistics supporting eugenics: "Better" families have too few children.[4]

problematic traits are "recessives" that can be passed along from parent to child without anyone really being bothered by them too deeply—kind of like complementary parts of a bomb. But if both mother and father carriers were to pass these traits on to the same child, the mechanisms of the heredity bomb would click into place, armed to explode.

The sad thing is, too few people have paid attention to this scientific information. And now civilization itself is on the cusp of disaster because of these sorts of people. To prevent this grand-scale collapse, we must work locally, individually, family by family, school by school, and hospital by hospital to identify the defective and eliminate them, while we simultaneously uplift the best examples among us. The unwanted humans—like rats and cockroaches—multiply faster than the good—at least if left unmanaged. And, ultimately, it's much more costly in tax dollars to support the undesirable. If we do nothing, the poor, the criminal, and the insane will overpopulate the earth, making it difficult for us normal folks to enjoy our status quo lives. Thankfully, we scientists and physicians have the tools to fix the situation, to disarm these genetic bombs, to even out the odds, if only governments would allow us to. What's more, these tools are not dangerous; they're part of good science and good medicine.

This was an international narrative. But, as the Second International Congress of Eugenics made it clear, a peculiarly Anglo-American framework scaffolded it. All the positive examples were white, heteronormative, wealthy, educated professionals from England and the American Northeast (New England), who exhibited a certain kind of manly pluck and womanly virtue. Immigrants, by and large, could not possess these positive values and, in fact, were far more likely to be

STATE EXPENSES FOR MAINTAINING STATE INSTITUTIONS FOR THE SOCIALLY INADEQUATE CLASSES, 1916.
(Not including county or other local expenditures.)

(From Statistical Dictionary of State Institutions for the Defective, Dependent and Delinquent Classes, Bureau of the Census, 1919.)

	Total	Rank among states	Per cent of total state expenditures for this purpose	Rank among states
Alabama	$ 425,018	40	5.4	48
Arizona	255,922	45	12.7	37
Arkansas	743,372	28	18.5	16
California	3,228,827	6	15.4	24
Colorado	684,053	31	18.1	17
Connecticut	1,503,022	14	20.5	10
Delaware	91,782	49	10.8	45
District of Columbia	315,280	41	3.5	49
Florida	491,854	36	16.2	22
Georgia	836,225	26	13.4	33
Idaho	279,667	43	14.9	29
Illinois	4,665,459	4	23.7	5
Indiana	2,578,716	8	14.4	30
Iowa	2,000,907	12	22.6	7
Kansas	1,404,173	16	24.3	3
Kentucky	1,339,818	17	13.4	32
Louisiana	933,902	23	13.2	27
Maine	753,372	27	10.9	43
Maryland	1,113,561	18	16.4	19
Massachusetts	6,322,275	2	30.5	1
Michigan	2,849,261	7	15.3	25
Minnesota	2,258,719	11	13.6	31
Mississippi	716,300	30	13.2	28
Missouri	1,885,125	13	20.0	11
Montana	589,949	34	16.1	18
Nebraska	976,516	22	23.4	6
Nevada	135,810	48	11.2	40
New Hampshire	456,840	39	22.2	8
New Jersey	2,311,680	9	13.3	34
New Mexico	186,453	46	11.6	39
New York	11,230,856	1	20.9	9
North Carolina	883,785	25	19.3	13
North Dakota	485,709	37	12.6	38
Ohio	3,966,756	5	24.6	2
Oklahoma	1,056,137	20	19.9	12
Oregon	621,676	33	16.3	21
Pennsylvania	4,772,212	3	15.2	26
Rhode Island	739,030	29	24.3	4
South Carolina	466,598	38	16.4	20
South Dakota	493,200	35	15.6	23
Tennessee	1,058,395	19	18.7	14
Texas	2,285,383	10	12.7	36
Utah	265,191	44	9.4	47
Vermont	287,011	42	16.3	46
Virginia	908,329	21	11.2	42
Washington	956,286	21	11.2	41
West Virginia	683,983	32	18.7	15
Wisconsin	1,111,576	15	10.9	41
Wyoming	165,261	47	12.8	35
Total	$75,203,239	Average	17.3	

Expense of state institutions for incarcerating the socially inadequate, according to *Eugenical News* (1919)

classified as "cacogenic." Americans of African or indigenous American descent didn't exist anywhere in this story, given the default, too-obvious-to-mention superiority of northern white European stock, as channeled by those who led and financially supported this eugenics congress.

To say that the American eugenics movement in the early twentieth century was an attempt to create a "master race," as some popular authors have done, is a bit of a caricature.[5] Theirs was not a *progressive* story prosecuted by liberal reformers, no matter how badly present-day conservatives in the US and the

UK want it to be.[6] Rather than trying to build anything new, the eugenics story was deeply *conservative* and *eliminative*: attempting to uphold the dominance of heteronormative elites against the onslaught of defectives, homosexuals, and lesser races. This belief is literally the *inverse* of so-called social Darwinism, which argued that the status quo must be left unmolested so that the politically and economically dominant can continue dominating. Instead, twentieth-century eugenicists clanged the same alarm bells rung in the nineteenth century by archconservatives like Gobineau and the Wagnerites: If you do nothing, if you refuse to tamper with reproduction, the ones you don't want will overwhelm and eventually replace you.

Major International Meetings

Dozens of regional meetings supplemented three major international eugenics congresses. Each one had a different flavor, and each meeting encouraged regional movements that fueled eugenics practices in nearly every corner of the globe. Of course, the meetings featured "great men," who delivered the major addresses. But more significant for the hidden history of eugenics, these meetings also spawned unnumerable unnamed "daily" eugenicists—the physicians and public health officials and bureaucrats who carried back to their communities the scientific messages about "the unfit" and the medical practices aimed at cutting off the lineages of degenerates. The powerful International Federation of Eugenics Organizations (IFEO), headed by Charles Davenport, stood behind many of these meetings and held its own organizational meetings every even-numbered year through the 1920s and '30s. But there were significant frenemy organizations that played an outsized role in spreading the eugenics word. The Latin International

Federation of Eugenics Organizations (LIFEO) began under the famous statistician Corrado Gini to counterbalance the US influence on the movement. Eventually including "non-Nordic" nations from southern and eastern Europe as well, LIFEO was interrupted by World War II but resumed until 1965, even after the IFEO dissolved.

The First International Eugenics Congress gathered almost four hundred top figures in eugenics, medicine, and politics at the Hotel Cecil in London from July 24 to 29, 1912. With Winston Churchill in the audience, Major Leonard Darwin delivered the keynote address connecting eugenics to his father's work revealing natural evolutionary laws. But American eugenicists argued the opposite: They wanted massive intervention. Interfering with the natural order, by sterilizing those undesirables with many children, would be the only way forward. A small number of Norwegian, Greek, and French eugenicists attended alongside the English, Canadians, and Americans who filled the event.

The Second International Congress, from September 25 to 27, 1921, outlined at the beginning of this chapter, completed the transfer of power away from "gentleman class" British eugenicists to middle-class professional American ones. The paleontologist H. F. Osborn hosted the meeting in New York. Madison Grant raised the funds and helped Harry Laughlin organize it. Alexander Graham Bell, inventor of the telephone, replaced Major Darwin as president. And even when Major Darwin did rise to speak, he now echoed the American line—marriage restrictions and elimination through sterilization. Bell joined in, too. Despite being the son and husband of deaf women, he argued for the elimination of deafness by means of eugenics. With the US State Department backing the congress and the Carnegie Foundation supplying funds for the AMNH exhibits and travel, the meeting attracted hundreds of visitors from all over the world. In addition to European and North American contingents (minus Germans, whom the French and British wouldn't allow), Argentina, Australia, Brazil, Colombia, Cuba, Japan, New Zealand, and several other nations sent delegates. Nevertheless, Americans dominated the space and gave nearly all the formal presentations, as one Swedish eugenicist loudly complained.[7]

The AMNH also hosted the Third International Eugenics Congress, from August 21 to 23, 1932. Once again, members from the American Eugenics Triangle dominated the organizing body and, therefore, delivered the talks. Major Leonard Darwin was now eighty-eight years old and could not attend. The entire British contingent could only manage to send a handful of representative eugenicists. Though the eugenics network now included Germans, Austrians, and other World War I enemies, Italian and Dutch participants submitted more scientific papers. Americans again clogged the program with almost fifty of the sixty-five papers. More South American, Caribbean, and Asian nations participated, however, indicating just how widespread and normal eugenics seemed even outside Anglo-American nations. As we'll see in a later chapter, attendees of this meeting would promote and organize "population control" activities in South America, Asia, and the Caribbean even after "eugenics" had become a dirty word, associated with the Nazis.

Financially, the eugenics movement appeared more robust than ever. The Harriman family railroad fortune, once again, financially backed the whole conference. Genetic data gathered from W. Averell Harriman's thoroughbred horses played a prominent role in the Third Congress's AMNH exhibits. (Aside from being one of the wealthiest men in America, Averell Harriman would soon go on to serve as US ambassador to the USSR during World War II, then ambassador to the UK, then Secretary of Commerce under President Harry S. Truman, then the forty-eighth governor of New York, and finally, Secretary of State for both President Kennedy and President Johnson.) Laughlin and Grant also roped in the blue-blooded fortunes of the Roosevelt, Dodge, Pratt, Draper, and du Pont Copeland families to support eugenics.

Interestingly, each decade's congress changed its emphasis slightly. Early on, degeneration, low white birthrates, and violent crime occupied eugenicists' minds. Later, disease, migration, and high birthrates of non-whites dominated. With very few exceptions, however, the master narrative about locating defects, eliminating those defects from the race, and excluding inferior races from dominating "white" nations remained constant from paper to exhibit, congress to congress.

Table of Sterilizations Done in State Institutions Under State Laws Up To and Including the Year 1940

| STATE | DIAGNOSIS AND SEX | | | | | | | | | SEX SUMMARY | | |
| | INSANE | | | FEEBLEMINDED | | | OTHERS | | | TOTALS | | |
	MALE	FEMALE	TOTAL	MALE	FEMALE	TOTAL	M.	F.	T.	MALE	FEMALE	TOTAL
ALA.	0	0	0	129	95	224	0	0	0	129	95	234
ARIZ.	10	10	20	0	0	0	0	0	0	10	10	20
CAL.	5,329	4,310	9,639	2,166	2,763	4,929	0	0	0	7,495	7,073	14,568
CONN.	19	337	356	6	56	62	0	0	0	25	393	418
DEL.	206	71	277	116	193	309	0	24	24	322	288	610
GA.	6	68	74	22	31	53	0	0	0	28	99	127
IDAHO	2	10	12	2	0	2	0	0	0	4	10	14
IND. A14	213	177	390	336	305	643	0	0	0	551	482	1,033
IOWA	83	91	174	25	121	146	4	12	16	112	234	336
KANS.	1,035	724	1,759	342	205	547	38	60	98	1,415	989	2,404
ME.	0	10	10	14	104	118	0	62	62	14	176	190
MICH.	71	234	305	417	1,324	1,741	25	74	99	513	1,632	2,145
MINN.	113	266	379	273	1,228	1,501	0	0	0	386	1,494	1,850
MISS.	135	320	455	14	42	56	0	12	12	149	374	523
MONT.	16	20	36	42	108	150	0	0	0	58	128	186
NEB.	53	90	143	101	144	245	0	0	0	154	234	388
N.H.	34	266	190	49	141	190	0	50	50	73	357	430
N.Y.	0	41	41	0	0	0	1	0	1	1	41	42
N.C.	90	150	240	93	538	631	42	104	146	225	792	1,017
N.D.	123	174	297	51	158	209	11	17	28	185	349	534
OKLA.	70	232	302	27	141	168	0	0	0	97	373	470
ORE.	287	321	608	235	506	741	30	71	101	552	898	1,450
S.C.	0	0	0	1	34	35	0	0	0	1	34	35
S.D.	0	0	0	206	354	560	6	11	17	212	365	577
UTAH	44	43	87	99	66	165	0	0	0	143	109	252
VER.	1	12	13	56	118	174	9	16	25	66	146	212
VA.	976	1,365	2,341	660	923	1,583	0	0	0	1,636	2,288	3,924
WASH.	141	245	386	33	242	275	4	2	6	178	489	667
W. Va.	0	18	18	0	9	9	1	18	19	1	45	46
WIS.	0	0	0	165	991	1,156	0	0	0	165	991	1,156
TOTALS:	9,047	9,505	18,552	5,682	10,940	16,622	171	533	704	14,900	20,978	35,878

Eugenics Around the World

International attendees of these congresses adapted that master narrative to their own cultural contexts. Ultimately, most major countries on every continent adopted eugenics measures. Non-Anglo eugenicists often disassociated their version of eugenics from the bigotry they felt emanating from American and British eugenicists. Yet all retained that focus on the heteronormative family: traditional masculine and feminine roles that translated to "enlightened reproduction."[8] Eugenicists labeled anything else sexual deviance, a target for intervention.

In truth, it is too easy for us today to wave our hands and discount eugenics as a pseudoscience safely encapsulated in the past. What I hope to impress upon you with this very circumscribed selection is just how quickly these ideas became pervasive across nation after nation—East and West, North and South, rich and poor, conservative and progressive.

Argentina

Under the National Direction of Maternity and Infancy, created in 1936, eugenicists pushed policies to encourage large families among the ideal "Argentinean biotype" and attempted endocrinological treatments to transform women into those ideal types.[9] A strongly Catholic country under a penal code ban on such practices, Argentina seemed to have very few sterilizations, or "negative" eugenics. Physicians later revealed that almost no doctors *publicly reported* sterilizations due to government oversight. Yet they occurred frequently.[10]

Australia

A. O. Neville, Chief Protector of Aborigines for Western Australia, and Dr. Cecil Cook, the Northern Territory Chief Protector, plus scores of their colleagues and successors all across Australia and the neighboring Torres Strait Islands, forcibly removed indigenous children from their parents from the 1920s through the '70s. "Protectors" hoped to resegregate races by "breeding white" the mixed-race children placed in white Australian "foster care"—it was that or fully racially segregating or sterilizing those unable to be bred white. "The problem of our half-castes," Cook explained, "will quickly be eliminated by the complete disappearance of the black race, and the swift submergence of their progeny in the white."[11] Neville's and Cook's policies proved so persuasive that prominent American eugenicists sought to emulate them: "Australia is handling the situation with great wisdom," reflected W. A. Plecker, an architect of the *Buck v. Bell* eugenics case, "by neither allowing miscegenation nor even permitting the migration of colored races to the country."[12] Perhaps as many as a third of indigenous families fell victim to this "Stolen Children" practice—the reason behind Australia's "National Sorry Days" beginning in 1998.[13]

Brazil

Joseph Arthur de Gobineau served as France's ambassador to Brazil from 1869 to 1870 and befriended Brazil's emperor, Dom Pedro II. Their relationship continued to have an impact on Brazil's trajectory following the emancipation of slavery in 1889. For the next quarter century, Brazil implemented a policy of "whitening" African blood out of the population—*branqueamento*—by attracting a massive immigration of Europeans. Physicians and reformers stirred up familiar fears about mixed race degenerate *mestiços* and strongly pushed sterilization and marriage restrictions in pursuit of "hygiene." In addition, like Anglo-American eugenicists, they attempted to restrict non-white immigration. This came to a head in the 1929 Eugenics Congress, the largest of its kind in South America—but also the only such meeting.

Unlike in the US or Germany, Brazilian eugenics in the period from 1920 to 1940 never fully adopted an anti-racial-minority cast. Opposition from the Catholic Church, anthropologists, and intellectuals behind the *Manifesto dos Intelectuais Brasileiros contra o Preconceito Racial* ("Manifesto of Brazilian Intellectuals Against Racism"), plus infighting among Brazilian eugenicists, successfully redirected eugenics policies toward improved environmental, educational, and health policy rather than surgeries.[14]

Canada

Just after the *Buck v. Bell* case in the US, and with the outspoken support of Emily Murphy, a suffragist and the first female magistrate of the British Empire, Alberta passed the Sexual Sterilization Act (1928). British Columbia and Saskatchewan followed. Eventually, Canadian eugenicists would coercively sterilize over three thousand people deemed "defective." As elsewhere, the blade fell most often upon racial minorities— First Nations, Métis people, and Eastern Europeans—as well as single, impoverished mothers, even if they showed no signs of disability. Those laws remained active until the 1970s.[15]

In 1996, Canadian courts ruled in favor of Leilani Muir, a woman sterilized without her knowledge at Alberta's Provincial Training School for Mental Defectives in 1959, when she was fifteen. Doctors at the time informed her that she had had an appendectomy. Muir's case launched a reexamination of Canada's past eugenics. In 1999, Alberta's provincial government formally apologized and offered around eighty-one million Canadian dollars to several hundred living victims of coerced sterilization under Canada's eugenics laws.[16]

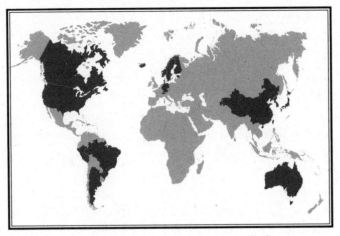

Nations with active eugenics programs in the first
half of the twentieth century; shaded nations had an active program

China

Though the first Chinese contingent in the international
eugenics movement didn't appear until 1932, Pan Guangdan
(Quentin Pan), a former student of Charles Davenport's,
became an influential proponent of eugenics in Republican China beginning in the 1920s. His books, articles, and
the journal *Eugenics Monthly*—later rebranded as *Huanian*,
meaning "helping the race reach maturity"—guided Chinese
government policies before and after World War II. China's
first explicitly eugenic marriage law appeared in 1950, banning
marriage between relatives or between those with certain diseases, like leprosy.[17]

Still, despite Pan's influence and the new concern with pre-
nuptial investigations of family genealogies to ensure healthy
offspring, Western ideas of genetic determinism never dominated. Pan also remained a critic of the racism he saw in Anglo-
American eugenics. In Maoist China, "eugenics" involved

marriage counseling and public health measures to combat syphilis, tuberculosis, alcoholism, opioid abuse, and the *mui-tsai* child trafficking system, rather than immigration restrictions or sterilizations.[18] Pan himself was condemned during the Cultural Revolution for reactionary views, including "population control" (more on that later). However, Communist Party insiders rehabilitated his legacy after his death, and a more Western-style eugenics began to spread in the 1970s.[19]

Japan

In 1911, Yamanouchi Shigeo, a distinguished young algae specialist at the University of Chicago, attended a series of lectures headlined by Charles Davenport. Upon his return to Japan in 1913, Yamanouchi borrowed from Davenport's recruitment skills to launch several eugenics organizations, including the Greater Japan Eugenics Society (Dai Nihon Yûseikai) in 1917. While the GJES didn't last long, its members became prominent advocates of marriage restrictions and, eventually, successfully pushed for the National Eugenic Law in 1940.[20] Among other things, the newly established eugenic marriage counseling centers set up by the law identified the precise anatomical measurements of the eugenically ideal Japanese man and woman and then offered this vague threat about racial hygiene and the war of races.

> For every Japanese child born, seven children are born in China, five in India, and three in the Soviet Union. However important it is to increase the population, the birth of physically weak and mentally impaired children will harm the national body. Therefore, let us be sure to think carefully about marriage and to transact a wholesome union in order to bring forth superior offspring.[21]

During World War II, physicians sterilized approximately five hundred people under this law. And these policies also had a lasting impact on Korean society, even after the Japanese occupation ended.

After the collapse of the Empire, the Japanese government under American supervision passed the Eugenic Protection Law in 1948. Aside from marriage restrictions, the law established a Eugenic Protection Commission to oversee involuntary sterilizations of the unfit—under which they included those with "remarkable criminal inclination." As the Ministry of Health and Welfare clarified in 1953, sterilizations could be "performed against a patient's will" employing even restraints and deception, provided the operating physician felt it necessary. Over the next half century, Japanese physicians enacted this eugenics law to involuntarily sterilize at least sixteen thousand people.[22]

Scandinavia

From 1922 to 1958, the Scandinavian peninsula—the heartland of Gobineau's, Grant's, Stoddard's, and others' mythological Aryanism—ran a robust eugenics program through Sweden's *Statens institut för rasbiologi* (State Institute for Racial Biology) at Uppsala University. Scandinavian geneticists and anthropologists braided their eugenics insights with their science from the very beginning of the twentieth century, predating even American involvement. And Swedish, Danish, Finnish, Icelandic, and Norwegian physicians and politicians stressed the importance of marriage restrictions and sterilizations far longer than most other European nations. Rather than overt racial motivations, however, Scandinavian eugenicists for the most part emphasized cost cutting measures.[23] By removing the hereditarily ill from the population, the welfare state could grow more robust for everyone else. Official counts put the number of sterilized in the name of eugenics at 175,000. But that number is under dispute, especially since fully voluntary sterilizations for birth control purposes were legalized almost as soon as eugenics practices officially ended in the mid-1970s.[24]

Switzerland

Switzerland never adopted a national eugenics program. Still, the 1912 Swiss Civil Code (ZGB) included provisions for publicly funded eugenic marriage counseling and made marriage illegal for those deemed mentally ill. And Otto Schlaginhaufen, a German-trained anthropologist and prolific measurer of skulls, remained a core member of the international eugenics movement throughout the 1930s. Aside from traditional political decentralization, Swiss eugenics never unified over the

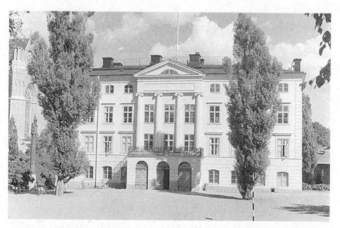

From 1922 to 1958, the Dekanhusset in Uppsala, Sweden, housed the successor to the Swedish Society for Racial Hygiene (1909–1921), as the Statens institut för rasbiologi (State Institute for Race Biology). The focus on human race and eugenics only ended after the 1960s.[25]

core issue of race. Antisemitism remained rampant and white supremacy a given in Swiss society in the first half of the century. Yet even Schlaginhaufen could not stomach the fascistic lurch to the right in the 1930s. When Ernst Rüdin, a eugenicist and a Nazi, presented the Third Reich's eugenics laws to Swiss psychiatrists in 1934, they scoffed. Only one Swiss canton (Vaud) ever established compulsory sterilization laws.

Yet a kind of soft eugenics persisted in medical clinics for decades. Beginning in the 1920s, medical providers adopted a policy of *junctim*. If a woman sought a legal abortion, physicians pressured her for sterilization, especially if doctors decided the woman was "unfit" for motherhood. Given the absence of legal guidance, the judgment of fitness was left entirely up to physicians. Few records indicate that physicians sterilized because of arguments about hereditary disease, degeneration, or racial hygiene. Instead, doctors listed "disorderly housekeeping" or "bad mothering" among their justifications for surgery. *Junctim* continued through the 1970s. And though never formalized as "eugenics," untold thousands of Swiss women report feeling social pressure to eliminate the possibility of future children who, because of illness, might raise the cost of the Swiss health care system.[26] Switzerland did not formally repudiate such practices until the 2000s.

Uruguay

Corporations, physicians, attorneys, and politicians aligned to create a "eugenic utopia" in Uruguay between the World Wars.[27] Rather than merely having a vision of eliminating degenerate heredity, Uruguayan psychiatrists and physicians called for a triad of interventions to benefit the whole nation (*note*: not just the white race). These interventions included

1) immigration screening to limit the sick and the old, 2) increased social welfare programs directed at children (Código del Niño), and 3) punitive and therapeutic interventions into alcoholism as the centerpiece of a broader public health effort. Isn't it interesting how none of these proposals sound anything like eugenics in the Euro-American contexts?

In fact, at the Second Pan American Conference of Eugenics and Homiculture, held in Buenos Aires in 1934, Uruguayan eugenicists explicitly rejected sterilization and racial explanations of degeneration. The three delegates from the US and their Latin American supporters attempted to get at least *voluntary* sterilization considered. They even read Harry Laughlin's contribution on degenerate Latin American races in support of their point. But the tone-deaf pushiness and racism of the North Americans only made the South American delegates angry. After this meeting, "eugenics" in Uruguay looked decidedly different than it did in the rest of the Euro-American sphere of influence.[28]

As this list demonstrates, by the beginning of the Great Depression, an international network of eugenicists encircled the globe. Though eugenics didn't look the same in every nation, the network's tendrils trailed across the medical and scientific landscape worldwide. British influence over this network

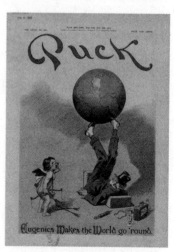

Eugenics Makes the World Go 'Round (1913)

slowly diminished, while the American Eugenics Triangle, from New York to California, strongly influenced similar practices from Tokyo to Cape Town to Buenos Aires. Soon, however, Germany eclipsed even the US's robust program, to become the central villain in the most notorious chapter in the history of eugenics.

CHAPTER 11

Making America White Again

Congressman Albert Johnson tapped Harry H. Laughlin, of New York's Eugenics Records Office, to give him scientific backing for his national plan to remake American immigration. In the name of eugenics, Johnson would pass draconian immigration policies in an attempt to make sure that the US would always remain a homeland for Grant's "great race." He couldn't have been prouder of the results. During World War II, for instance, the Johnson–Reed Act severely limited Jewish entrants into the US at the very moment Nazi persecution intensified—all part of the grand, global quest to clean the white race.

A Republican representing Washington's Third District, Johnson had grown up in the Midwest, like Laughlin, and worked as a journalist in New Haven, Connecticut, before moving to Tacoma. In 1913, he rode to local fame as an opinionated media firebrand (editor of the *Grays Harbor Washingtonian*). He may have twisted the truth a lot, but the louder and angrier his media tirades, the more powerful he became, eventually shouting his way into national politics. Johnson also possessed that politician's shape-shifting skill that allowed him to dance from one popular political position to its opposite, and to defend them with equal vehemence if his most influential constituents changed their minds. He retained his seat through ten congressional elections.

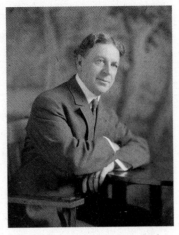

Albert Johnson (R-Washington)

On one topic, however, Johnson would not be moved regardless of public opinion: Johnson couldn't stand immigrants. Thankfully for him, his white constituents always agreed. He channeled the fears enunciated by Grant and Stoddard about the "Yellow Peril" threatening to replace whites. East Asian expats—whom he quietly employed as his own domestic servants—especially irked politician Johnson. It's true that he saw how his fellow whites mistreated the foreigners: "The coolies were penned up, treated like peons, and herded away to work on the section gangs of the railroads." It's just that he didn't see inhumanity as the problem: "*Inducements* were offered to bring those Japanese laborers here."[1] He used his media and then his political platforms to scream about the existence of non-whites rather than their treatment at the hands of whites. And his audience grew and grew.

Though a pro-business Republican, Johnson joined with Washington state's Asiatic Exclusion League and claimed to be among the five-hundred-man mob of blue-collar white laborers who hounded other blue-collar South Asian laborers out of Bellingham, Washington, and into Canada in September 1907.[2] Johnson titled the defining speech that launched him into the political elite *The Defense of Alaska—the Union of the White Race and the Problem of Universal Peace* (1913). In it, he laid out in no uncertain terms both his hope for a pure Caucasian ethnostate and his plans to attain it. He never owned up to donning the white robes of the Ku Klux Klan, the membership of which surged in the Northwest through the 1920s. Yet he never deviated from his rabid support for white supremacy, and the Klan rewarded him for it. They repeatedly made Johnson's reelection a pillar of the KKK's political platform—the only member of Congress to repeatedly and proudly accept that "honor."[3]

> "I take my stand [for Pan-aryanism] on the proposition that the terrible struggle for existence, produced in most parts of Asia . . . ought not to be communicated to other lands. . . . The question of Asiatic immigration is a question of life and death to the white race."
>
> —Albert Johnson, speech before the
> House of Representatives (1913)[4]

After two terms in Congress, and despite no knowledge of chemistry, Johnson became a captain in the new Chemical Warfare Service for a few months during World War I (though there is no evidence he ever left his DC office). Upon his return to civilian duties, he exchanged this military cachet for his holy grail: chairmanship of the House Committee on Immigration and Naturalization. From this position, he could stop non-whites from entering the country in the first place.

Johnson saw a natural ally in the eugenicist Harry H. Laughlin. The sentiment proved mutual. In a quid pro quo that resonated for a generation, Johnson used Laughlin's scientific justification to exclude those who, he asserted, were *biologically* unable to assimilate into white American Protestant Christian culture. Laughlin, in turn, used Johnson to raise awareness of feeblemindedness and moral insanity among non-whites and to inject eugenicists' wishes about widely applied genital surgery (relatively unpopular) into the national conversation vilifying immigrants (quite popular).

In 1921, the House Committee on Immigration and Naturalization, with key assistance from Laughlin and publicity from Madison Grant, successfully shepherded immigration restrictions never before seen in American society through Congress and the White House. Johnson's committee formulated the Emergency Quota Act, originally pitched by the Dillingham Commission in 1910. But instead of the lighter restrictions favored by Dillingham, Albert Johnson called for a "total and complete shutdown" of immigration into the US—until his group could figure out "what the hell was going on."[5]

Corporate interests in Johnson's Republican party disliked the downstream effects of this policy on their low-cost workforce. So, eventually Johnson compromised on annual quotas for each country of origin to 3 percent of the total number of foreign-born persons recorded in the 1910 census, strongly favoring Europeans and excluding almost all Asians and Africans. Bigot though he was, even President Woodrow Wilson opposed the bill for standing in the way of the attempt to rebuild international cooperation in the wake of the Great War. However, Wilson's successor, Warren G. Harding, a Republican, held no such scruples. He called a special session of Congress to pass the Emergency Quota Act and, as soon as the newly elected president signed it, forced ports to literally turn boats around and send immigrants back out to sea.

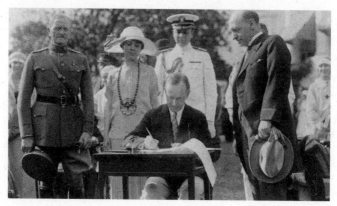

President Calvin Coolidge signs the anti-immigration
Johnson–Reed Act in 1924.

In contrast to the eight hundred thousand immigrants that
arrived in 1920, barely three hundred thousand made it in
1922.[6]

Still, Johnson remained dissatisfied. In 1924, he made
the connection between white supremacy and eugenics aim
of eliminating the "unfit" more explicitly than any American with such political power ever had. Johnson's committee
teamed up with Senator David Aiken Reed, the new conservative face from Pittsburgh, to craft the even more draconian
Johnson–Reed Act. Because of their work, almost no one
deemed unfit—whether because of hereditary defect, Jewish
faith, or their lack of whiteness—would find refuge in the
US. Immigration plunged from even 1922's 300,000 to barely
150,000 annually. And of that reduced number, over 100,000
originated in white enclaves of northern Europe.

The political revolution that took place in the wake of the
Great Depression finally unseated Johnson. Still, the eugenics
legacy he built with Laughlin's scientific scaffolding continued
to exclude unwanted immigrants as the country turned away

thousands of Eastern European Jews fleeing the Nazi grinder. For forty years, America basically shut the door entirely to Africans, Asians, Pacific Islanders, and other non-whites, until the civil rights movement pried it open.

> "There is today one state in which at least weak beginnings toward a better conception [of immigration] are noticeable. Of course, it is not our model German Republic, but the United States."
>
> —Adolf Hitler[7]

Laughlin hailed the Johnson–Reed Act as a substantial victory for racial purity, and it would be hard not to hear echoes of that policy through the rest of the century and

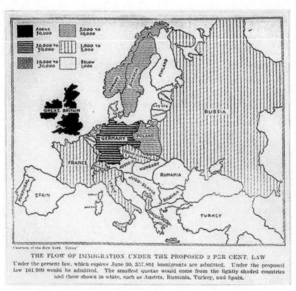

The Johnson–Reed Act immigration restriction hoped to refocus the population flow on those traditional "Aryan" nations.

beyond. For instance, in a 2015 radio interview, Trump's nominee for attorney general, Jeff Sessions, praised the 1924 Johnson–Reed Act. Stopping the immigration of non-whites and assimilating those deemed to fit within the eugenicists' vision of the US created the "solid middle class of America," claimed Sessions.[8] When President Johnson helped overturn that legislation in 1965, it opened the door to non-whites. And by the twenty-first century, Sessions lamented that America was "on a path to surge far past what the situation was in 1924." Making America great again, Sessions implied on-air, would mean going back to the anti-white quotas of the 1920s.

Ironically, the "Nordics" of Norway, Sweden, Iceland, Denmark, and the Netherlands—who Representative Albert Johnson and his comrades in white robes *wanted* to immigrate—also substantially reduced their once robust demographic flow into the US after Johnson–Reed. And this, perhaps more than any newfound love for racial and ethnic diversity, may have helped Congress lift the restrictions in the mid-1960s.[9]

CHAPTER 12

Nazi Ties

In the history of science and race and eugenics, all roads lead to the Nazis. But this isn't just some corollary of Godwin's Law, in which every long, heated argument ends up comparing someone to the Nazis.[1] Almost unanimously and automatically, Nazis come to mind at the mere mention of race science or eugenics. At some gut level, we associate the most loathsome practices humans have ever conjured with Hitler's Germany. That has become part of the problem: We know almost *too much* about Nazis and eugenics. Hollywood and pop culture have amplified their heinousness (into zombie conjuring, for instance), and they have made Nazi physicians something alien—unlike regular folks like us. But of course, the vast machinery of the Holocaust, though orchestrated by villains like Hitler, Goebbels, Mengele, and Göring, had to be switched on and run day after day by regular people, some of whom were otherwise smart, accomplished, responsible, put-together, hardworking, even "nice."

The menace of Nazi eugenics differed less than we'd like to admit from the decades-long buildup of domestic and international policies and prejudices in other countries—even countries that fought the Nazis and liberated the camps. Sure, German science had its own distinctive trajectory. At the same time, German *Rassenhygiene* (race hygiene/cleaning) borrowed heavily from British and especially American scientists, physicians, and demagogues to stitch together the sentiments, statistics, and even the terminology deployed through the 1930s and '40s. Lothrop Stoddard's "under-man" label translated easily into *Untermensch* and rolled out across Germany in eugenics propaganda leaflets. The American biologist Joseph Graves put it best decades later: The road to Auschwitz-Birkenau ran through the Eugenics Records Office in Cold Spring Harbor, New York.[2]

Beyond that—and this is perhaps the worst news—the elimination of the Third Reich did not immediately or permanently dissolve beliefs that Nazis perpetuated and honed in their clinics attached to concentration camps. Many of the ideas about Jews, immigrants, the disabled, and dark-skinned people that we tie to the rise and fall of the Third Reich were revived, undead and lurching, into our contemporary policies and even daily lives. But we'll deal with that aftermath later.

We may never be able to answer the question that troubles us most: How do ideas about the relatedness—or differences—of groups of humans ever grow into the Frankensteinian monster of systematic genocide? Even if we can't answer the question, we should still be willing to trace the threads that, when woven together, became the fabric of the unspeakable.

Connecting with the Enemy

By the early 1920s, over the objections of Major Leonard Darwin, Britain's eugenics chief, Charles Davenport established a Permanent International Eugenics Commission. It first convened in Brussels, Belgium, with Alfred Ploetz, Erwin Baur, Fritz Lenz, and Eugen Fischer—the Big-Four scions of eugenics in Germany—in attendance. By the beginning of 1922, a renewed postwar movement to improve human breeding, under the moniker "eugenics," seemed assured. But then everything Davenport had worked for suddenly unraveled.

As part of the 1919 Versailles peace terms at the end of World War I, Germany agreed to give up the Rhineland, with the condition that no African-French troops be stationed there. But upholding promises to Senegalese leaders who bled for the Allied cause meant that the French government allowed a small number of soldiers from Senegal and North Africa to march into the Rhineland alongside the rest of the French army. German right-wing groups responded by protesting about the "black savages" presently descending upon helpless German women. Over 1920 and 1921, the British journalist Edmund D. Morel and the American actress Ray Beverage trumpeted fears to American, British, and German audiences that hypersexualized Africans would rape white women, and that French occupiers would look the other way, since this was another twist of the knife against their defeated German foe. The "Black Horror" or "Black Disgrace on the Rhine," they dubbed it. French degeneration due to racial crossbreeding would spread to Aryan Germany—just as Gobineau had decried a generation earlier. Their propaganda was so effective that mass protests erupted on the streets as far away as New York and London calling on France to pull out their Senegalese soldiers.[3]

In 1922, Germany defaulted on its coal and timber payments mandated by the Versailles Treaty. In response, Allied forces containing a relatively small number of non-white soldiers pushed farther east to occupy the Ruhr mining region in January 1923.[4] Predictably, cries of racial mixing in cities like Bochum, Dortmund, and Essen rang out. "Die schwarze Pest!"

and "Schwarze Schmach!" ("The Black Plague" and "Black Disgrace"), eugenicists screamed again in books, pamphlets, and newspaper articles distributed all across Europe and America.[5] Angry German eugenicists decided they wouldn't cooperate with the British, French, and Americans and pulled away from Davenport's eugenics network, leaving the other eugenicists to carry their torch on their own. Unde-

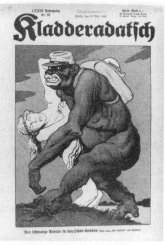

Ironically, racism—*Der Schwarze Terror* ("The Black Terror")—slowed international eugenics cooperation for a brief moment.

terred, Davenport chased them down one by one, again.

In the meantime, members of the Eugenics Triangle convinced the Canadians, the Scandinavian countries, Hungary, Poland, the Baltic countries, Czechoslovakia, Switzerland, and several other nations to take Germany's place in the eugenics movement. However, despite being home to Galton, who originated the term, and despite establishing the first university center for eugenics at University College London, Britain moved in the opposite direction by only reluctantly passing asylum legislation and shying away from sterilizations. (By the 1940s, the most stalwart British eugenicists, who were also some of the UK's best-known geneticists, lamented their "mild and flabby" eugenics program.[6]) In the first half of the 1920s, the Germans resolutely stood apart, excluded from this eugenics group. For a time, it seemed as if a truly robust international eugenics movement might never come to pass.

But by the middle of the decade Davenport could proudly hail the 1924 Johnson–Reed anti-immigration act, Virginia's anti-miscegenation law (banning interracial marriages), Grant's *The Passing of the Great Race* (1916), and Stoddard's books *The Rising Tide of Color* (1920) and *The Revolt Against Civilization* (1922) as examples of America's commitment to truly serious, race-based eugenics. With this, Davenport finally reeled the Germans back in. If eugenicists' commitment to white supremacy wasn't clear enough before, perhaps these indicators—and Davenport's doggedness—did the trick.

In the midst of all this international tumult, other forces were working within Germany to make racial issues more prominent in politics. Julius Friedrich Lehmann, a wealthy publisher of eugenics and psychiatry literature in Switzerland and Germany, came across an English copy of Grant's *Passing of the Great Race* in the early 1920s. When Lehmann read Grant's explanation of the "racial basis of European history," and then Stoddard's extension into global politics, a light bulb went on in his head. With Aryans under threat, Lehmann deduced, any measure to withhold the sterilizing knife from the criminal and defective, the "weakling" and "worthless race types," would eventually bring about the end of civilization. Grant and Stoddard provided Lehmann with seemingly scientific language to describe what he had been looking for: the history of and justification for surgically purifying the white race.

To promote these ideas as widely as possible in German-speaking Central Europe, Lehmann launched the "Thule Society," a secretive cabal, built in some cases on the foundations of Gobineau Society groups, that gradually helped push Adolf Hitler and the German Workers Party to power.[7] He pumped out propaganda attributing Germany's losses in World War I to race degeneration, the machinations of Jews, and the spread of perfidious Marxism. Lehmann placed these pamphlets conspicuously in doctors' offices and hospital waiting rooms, where returning soldiers or their grieving

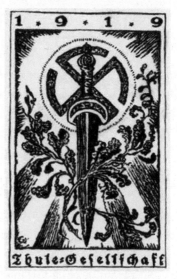

Julius Friedrich Lehmann's "Thule Society"

family members might read them. Lehmann also rushed to have his press promote a new German translation of Grant's *Passing of the Great Race*. He then took over the editorship of *Archiv für Rassen und Gesellschaftsbiologie* ("Archive for Race & Sociobiology") and *Volk und Rasse* ("People and Race"), adding respected scientific journals to the swelling river of white supremacist literature increasingly visible across Germany in the 1920s.[8]

By 1927, running behind the wave of Lehmann's propaganda, and with the *Buck v. Bell* trial making international news, Davenport finally tied up the international threads and founded the influential International Federation of Eugenics Organizations (IFEO). They set their first meeting in Geneva in 1934 to bring Germans into the official, scientific fold. Davenport also tapped Eugen Fischer to lead the special IFEO commission on race mixing and degeneration.

Fischer was a legend in German scientific and eugenics circles before the 1920s and was the natural choice to lead such a commission. His experience included acting as a race-mixing Grand Inquisitor in German-occupied Southwest Africa (Namibia) before and during World War I. In this region, German soldiers exterminated tens of thousands of Nama and Herrero people in concentration camps—a full generation before using such camps again in Central Europe.[9] In the years between 1923 and 1927, Fischer rose to become head of the brand-new Kaiser Wilhelm Institute of Anthropology, Human Heredity, and Eugenics. As head of the Institute, he also had access to one of the world's largest collections of skulls and preserved brains, including scores of samples stolen from southwest Africa. That skull collection became the cornerstone of the growing eugenics movement's textbook

in Germany: *Principles of Human Heredity and Race Hygiene*, by Erwin Baur, Eugen Fischer, and Fritz Lenz, with five editions between 1921 and 1940.

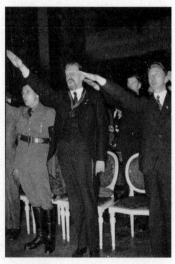

Eugen Fischer, a German anthropologist and central eugenics figure, at a Nazi rally in 1934

Principles ended up in the hands of Adolf Hitler, along with propaganda on race mixing, degeneration, and eugenics from Lehmann's press, including the works of Grant and Stoddard.[10] Tellingly, samplings of these publications are all over *Mein Kampf.*

Hitler also appreciated the work of one of Fischer's students, Hans F. K. Günther, whose *German Racial Types* (1922) turned out to be another bestseller for Lehmann.

A ten-man delegation of Nazi eugenicists, calling themselves "race hygienists" and copiously quoting Fischer and Günther, attended Davenport's first IFEO congress and immediately made their presence felt. A year later, in 1935, some of the same individuals appeared at the World Population Congress of the International Union for the Scientific Investigation of Population Problems (IUSIPP), held in Berlin. During the 1930s and '40s, "population control" was intertwined with white supremacist eugenics thought, but after World War II only partially disentangled itself from the movement, as we'll see below.

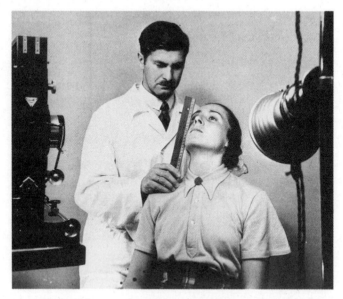

The facial features of a young German woman are measured
during a racial examination.

The future looked bleak, admitted the Nazi scientists at the IUSIPP in 1935, but solutions stood right in front of them. Whether called "eugenics" or "race hygiene" or the new popular term "population control," Germany—all of Europe, really—needed to stop merely pontificating and wringing their hands over the already occurring degeneration of civilization and truly follow the trail blazed by American physicians for eliminating the undesirable. Without drastic action, warned one German eugenicist steeped in the literature coming out of America, "white peoples would die out."[11]

CHAPTER 13

To Murder Six Million

Frank Capra's classic film *It Happened One Night* debuted in 1936. So did the toe-tapping Ginger Rogers and Fred Astaire blockbuster *Swing Time*. But that same year, many schools and churches across the US showed radically different sorts of films to thousands of adults and children. These movies were silent, featuring no movie stars—just a pastiche of grainy, quick cuts of buildings and ordinary people going about their lives. *Das Erbe* ("The Inheritance," 1935) and *Erbkrank* ("The Hereditary Defective," 1936) were two of the most often shown; both were produced by the Nazi propaganda machine.[1] Harry H. Laughlin had brought them to America and, drawing from the deep pockets of the American fascist Wickliffe Draper (whom we'll meet again below) and other blue-blooded supporters of the international eugenics congresses, took them on tour.[2]

The opening scene of *The Hereditary Defective* depicts small children playing outside a tenement in a large city— it could be New York or London or Berlin. "Criminals and morons build palaces for the descendants of drunkards, while workers and peasants have to make do with sorrowful hovels," reads an intertitle. In another scene, a park contains a dozen middle-aged women, smiling and talking. But there's something not quite right about the way they move about. One approaches the cameraman, upset at being filmed. "Jewish people have a particularly high percentage of intellectual freaks," the film explains as it pans over the group. In yet another, orderlies walk a line of smiling, mentally disabled children toward an asylum. "The rise of the mentally ill has increased 450 percent in the past seventy years," intertitles warn, and "in about fifty years there would be one mentally insane person for every four healthy people." More information flashes across the screen about how drunks, degenerates, and criminals cost the taxpayer an ungodly sum of money. For a time, the film explains, a universal struggle for survival culled their number. But now, misplaced Christian charity supports them and, worse, allows them to breed! Forced sterilization of these "useless eaters" would restore a natural balance—and allow citizens to keep more of their money. Throughout the films, patriotism and trust in science cloak the appeals to self-interest and fear of undesirables. "Practical love for one's neighbor," as *The Hereditary Defective* reinterprets the Golden Rule, "is in the prevention of genetically ill offspring."

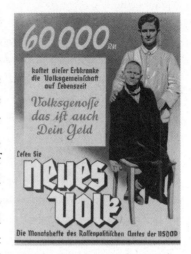

Nazi propaganda poster decrying the high cost of keeping a mentally ill person alive: "Comrades, that is also your money," the poster proclaimed unsubtly (c. 1937).

The American children, teachers, parents, principals, pastors, and civic leaders who watched Laughlin's Nazi propaganda had perhaps encountered similar messages at state fairs or eugenics demonstrations in museums. But in Germany, now under the control of propagandists like Joseph Goebbels, old degeneration fears and eugenics promises became fresh cultural narratives couched as morality tales. *Opfer der Vergangenheit: Die Sünde wider Blut und Rasse* ("Victims of the Past: The Sin Against Blood and Race," 1937) rivaled the quality of Leni Riefenstahl's more famous propaganda films and earned Hitler's highest praise. *Ich klage an* ("I Accuse," 1941), a moving, Hollywood-quality film in which a wife suffering from illness asks for euthanasia and is nearly denied by her pious husband, premiered under spotlights in Berlin and appeared in all German cinemas. (Clint Eastwood's 2004 critically acclaimed film *Million Dollar Baby* took many cues from *Ich klage an*, including a moving match of the final euthanasia scene.) *Why should the state care for the useless or permit the degenerated to reproduce?* these films asked. Wouldn't it be better for civilization, for the white race, for the taxpayer—and more merciful, more *Christian*—to stop the bad from breeding or even to euthanize the imperfect if they or their family or a kindly, competent physician thought it best for everyone? It was, of course, a decades-old message by now. Only these propaganda films were not merely showcasing the scientific message about heredity and degeneration. They were cover for borrowed eugenic medical techniques.

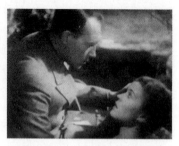

Euthanasia scene from *Ich klage an* ("I Accuse," 1941)

Behind the scenes, race hygienists and their physician colleagues in Germany, Austria, the Czechoslovakian Sudetenland, and

Poland were already putting these sentiments—promoted for decades but deployed only in America and only in part—into terrifyingly efficient practice.

Aktion T-4

Historians have written mountains of books and essays on the inhumanities of German National Socialism (Nazism) during the Holocaust. Yet the eugenics movement that preceded the European death camps is still underrecognized. In the summer of 1933, within the first few months of Hitler's term as chancellor, Germany instituted a Prevention of Hereditarily Diseased Offspring law. Written largely by Ernst Rüdin, who attended Davenport's eugenics congresses, the law closely resembled Harry Laughlin's Model Sterilization Law. In truth, the German law was *less* restrictive than the American model; as written and practiced by American eugenicists, criminals and moderate drinkers were subject to sterilization surgery as well. The Nazi judicial system would continue to borrow and modify American anti-immigration and pro-racial segregation legislation throughout the 1930s.[3] With their version of eugenics, however, Germany created a streamlined system that American decentralization could never sustain. The propaganda films played a central part in justifying and mobilizing their legal and medical efforts.

> "Germany in a few months outdistanced California's sterilization world record of a quarter-century. . . . We must study Germany's methods."
> —Charles M. Goethe, a California real estate magnate and founder of California State University, Sacramento, in a speech to the Sacramento Twenty-Third Club (1938)[4]

Between 1934 and 1944, the Third Reich spawned nearly two hundred Hereditary Health Courts to adjudicate sterilization cases. Two physicians schooled in eugenics plus a judge drawn from the local magistrate court rigorously ran each one. The process of appeal proved to be straightforward and, unlike in American cases, many of those ordered to be sterilized did successfully appeal.[5] Lothrop Stoddard, whose *Rising Tide of Color* (1920) contributed to this mess in the first place, sat in on a session of one such health court.[6] Within the first two years of the German eugenics program, surgeons had sterilized more men and women than the American eugenicists had in twenty; by the early-1940s, that figure topped four hundred thousand.[7]

> "[Regarding] human trash in the big cities, certainly one million [could be] shoveled aside."
> —Ernst Bergmann, German philosopher[8]

But even that process seemed inefficient to those in power. After all, as eugenicists had been saying for decades, degenerates were here now. And their care cost a great deal of money. In 1938, as Hitler and his henchmen readied for war, the National Socialists decided to cut expenses, like good capitalists would. Their strategy was to declare internal war against the weak. When Stoddard visited the Grenadierstrasse in Berlin (now Almstadtstrasse in Berlin's Mitte district) in search of such "human trash" during his 1940 examination, he found nearly all the inhabitants were Eastern European Jewish immigrants. Stoddard understood why the neighborhood's residents looked "fear-ridden, sullen" under the Nazis but did not disagree with a postal carrier who spat, "All sorts of trash live here!" This was, the widely read Stoddard reported to his American audience, a perfectly rational reaction.

> *The relative emphasis which Hitler gave racialism and eugenics many years ago foreshadows the respective interest toward the two subjects in Germany today. . . . Inside Germany, the Jewish problem is regarded as a passing phenomenon, already settled in principle and soon to be settled in fact by the physical elimination of the Jews. . . . It is the regeneration of the Germanic stock with which public opinion is most concerned and which it seeks to further in various ways.*[9]

Stoddard wrote this in 1940, two years before "The Final Solution"—the euphemistic term used by Nazi leaders about the systemic mass murder of European Jews. What he could not know is that Hitler had already consented to a national extermination quota proposed by his inner circle. Their justification was simple: bad lives, which cost society money, would need to be sacrificed to offset the biological cost of good lives lost in combat.

Sterilization in the 1930s soon gave way to out-and-out mass murder in the "Euthanasia Movement" by 1940. Supposedly, this occurred because of a single piece of correspondence. In the spring of 1939, parents from a farm outside Leipzig petitioned Hitler directly to have their disabled infant, Gerhard Kretschmar, euthanized. Reich lawyers doubted such an order was legal—in addition to being patently immoral. But Hitler approved the request and physicians followed through. In microcosm, the death of baby Gerhard was the action all those decades of work promoted by eugenicists had been leading up to. Poor parents *appealing* to doctors to eliminate their defective child in order to keep him and their lineage from becoming a burden on the more fortunate! This was a

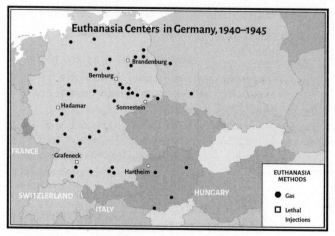

Euthanasia Centers in Germany, 1940–1945

Brandenburg

Bernburg

Hadamar

Sonnestein

FRANCE

Grafeneck

Hartheim

SWITZERLAND

HUNGARY

ITALY

EUTHANASIA
METHODS

● Gas

□ Lethal
Injections

Aktion T-4 centers euthanized patients throughout Germany and occupied territories prior to the Holocaust.

eugenics beyond the most hopeful imaginings of Plato, Gobineau, Woodhull, Galton, Reverend McCulloch, Grant, Stoddard, Davenport—even Laughlin.

But, just as in the US, the eugenics cyclone continued to spin faster and faster. The "trial balloon" of the Kretschmar case effectively launched a massive program of *Gnadentod* ("mercy killings") of the mentally and physically handicapped. From their offices on Tiergartenstrasse 4 ("T-4") in Berlin, Philip Bouhler, manager of the chancellery (chief of staff), and Dr. Karl Brandt, Hitler's personal physician—supported by the psychiatrists Werner Heyde and Paul Nitsche, biologists Kurt Pohlisch and Ernst Rüdin, along with three dozen health care workers—ordered the systematic killing of anyone deemed *Lebensunwertes Leben* ("life not worthy of life").

At first, physicians, nurses, and caretakers left victims, including thousands of German children, to starve in asylums. They claimed lethal injections were too expensive to fulfill the execution quota of one hundred thousand that Aktion T-4 (as later tribunals dubbed it) was supposed to fulfill. But starvation took too long. They tried piping automobile and bus exhaust into basements. Still, the process proved too slow, and the cries of the asphyxiating too distressing for staff and people in the neighborhood who could overhear the executions. Finally, they converted psychiatric hospitals into mass execution centers. At Bernburg, Brandenburg, Grafeneck, Hadamar, Hartheim, and Sonnenstein in Germany, and Am Spiegelgrund and Gugging in Austria, ordinary psychiatrists, physicians, and nurses, who had spent the majority of their careers caring for the ill, woke up, got dressed, ate breakfast, went from their homes to their jobs day after day, and chose to release lethal pesticide gases into basement "showers" where they had gathered their patients. (Newly developed Zyklon, created in the laboratory of Fritz Haber, the famed Jewish chemist and inventor of chlorine gas warfare in World War I, proved most effective. A few months later, Zyklon-B would be used to murder millions in Central European death camps, including many in Haber's family.) By the close of the war, German eugenicists had exceeded their goals, exterminating around one hundred thousand institutionalized people inside Germany and at least that many in conquered territories.[10] Few concerned citizens raised any objections about the elimination of the "unfit."

Punishing and Rehabilitating

When, at the end of the Moscow Conference in October 1943, Roosevelt and Stalin signed Churchill's condemnation of Nazi war crimes titled the "Statement on Atrocities," they cited "cold-blooded mass executions" and "wholesale shooting of Polish officers."[11] The highly publicized Nuremberg Trials wrapped up in the autumn of 1946, with twelve members of

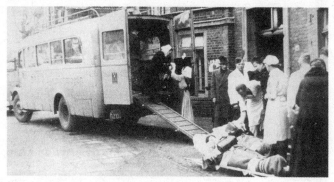

Bus transports unfit psychiatric patients to asylums as part of Aktion T-4

the Reich sentenced to death. But no one at any of these events mentioned the heinous acts committed in the name of science and medicine.

Then, in the winter of 1946 to 1947, the Nuremberg courtroom opened a second time for the case *United States of America v. Karl Brandt, et al.*, also known as the "Doctors' Trial" or the "Medical Case." It was the first of roughly a dozen additional trials, overseen exclusively by American justices and prosecutors, stretching late into 1948, that sought justice for the individuals American legal professionals believed were the worst administrators and financial supporters of the Holocaust.[12] Finally, Nazi eugenics would receive its comeuppance. Prosecutors regarded Hitler's physician, Karl Brandt, as the symbolic key to the rhetoric of justice surrounding the Doctors' Trial. Twenty-two other defendants, rounded up by Allies after the collapse of the Third Reich, joined Brandt. But Dr. Joseph Mengele, famous for inhumane twin-studies at Auschwitz-Birkenau, escaped capture and was never brought to trial. The tribunal accused the physicians of experimentation on live subjects, including rapid depressurization, burning with napalm, testing with experimental drugs, and intentional infection with painful and deadly diseases.

All that was gruesome, to be sure. But, once again, "eugenics" never appeared on the list of indictments. The charges spoke instead of acts done to noncombatants from other nations—without a word about the moral reclassification and dehumanization that allowed the subjects that were treated as lab rats in the first place. More than one of the German defendants noted with bitterness that their medical interventions, now labeled war crimes, were similar if not identical to medical trials conducted on prisoners and inmates of asylums in Allied countries. Judges insisted German experiments were illegal because the patients could not credibly give their consent. *Ah*, the Nazi defendants charged back, *but wasn't that exactly what was being done in America as part of the eugenics movement?* Wasn't this whole Doctors' Trial just another example, not of the righteous prosecution of internationally recognized moral codes, but of "might makes right"? German doctors stood trial because Allied armies marched into Berlin instead of Germans marching into London or Washington, DC. The American tribunal justices—and they were all Americans—passed over such paradoxes largely without comment.

Certainly, the German experiments deserved the strongest condemnation. But other troubling aspects slithered away from the American justices' attention. For instance, a number of laboratories and clinics throughout Europe rapidly

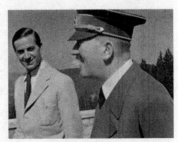

Dr. Karl Brandt with his patient,
Adolf Hitler, c. 1942

emerged from the ravages of war with greatly augmented collections of skulls and brains. Where did those new samples come from? Prominent scientific papers published after the war addressed the so-called "nature–nurture debate" regarding genetic differences in response to extremes of disease, starvation, or pain using twins. How were these twin studies conducted? The Nuremberg Trials have long been credited with dispensing justice without exacting unprofitable vengeance. Historians view that claim with some skepticism, however, and not just because the scientific enablers escaped trial for profiting from the carnage. In too many cases, the experimental work that emerged from Holocaust-enhanced collections became *mainstream* science, with those behind Aktion T-4 and the rest rehabilitated as ordinary physicians and scientists.

Take, for example, the eugenics-inspired twin studies conducted by Dr. Mengele at Auschwitz-Birkenau. Sure, the *experiments*—where one twin was the control and the

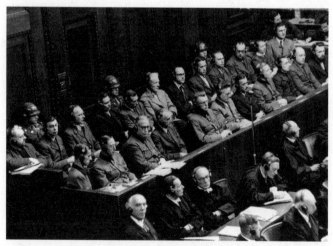

Nuremberg Doctors' Trial

other was subjected to heinous medical interventions—garnered outrage. But figures affiliated with Mengele's unethical studies hid in plain sight. Otmar Freiherr von Verschuer, for instance, Mengele's mentor. Verschuer directed the Institute for Genetic Biology and Racial Hygiene from 1935 to 1942, then the Kaiser Wilhelm Institute of Anthropology, Human Heredity, and Eugenics (KWI-A) from 1942 to 1948. He was an active participant at IFEO eugenics meetings and IUSIPP population control congresses through the 1930s and '40s. Verschuer procured many of Mengele's specimens during and after the internments, and he continued to practice human genetic studies unhindered for decades, even retaining organs taken from Auschwitz victims.[13] By the early 1950s, several prominent geneticists, including Ronald A. Fisher, a British follower of Galton and one of the lauded founders of the Modern (neo-Darwinian) Synthesis, successfully lobbied for Verschuer's rehabilitation.[14]

> "My assistant, Dr. Mengele (MD, PhD) has joined me in this branch of research. He is presently employed . . . at Auschwitz. Anthropological investigations on the most diverse racial groups of this concentration camp are being carried out with permission of the SS Reichsführer [Himmler]; the blood samples are being sent to my laboratory for analysis."
>
> —Otmar von Verschuer (1943)[15]

By the following decade, Verschuer had managed to shake off all Nazi associations and rebuild old networks. He continued his interest in population control and easily embedded himself within the International Association for the

Advancement of Ethnology and Eugenics (IAAEE), an organization that continued to be generously funded by Wickliffe Draper, a prominent American funder of eugenics before the war. And just a few years later, in 1961, partly as a reaction against *Brown v. Board of Education of Topeka, Kansas* (1954)—the Supreme Court case that began to undo generations of racial segregation in public schools—Verschuer and six other eugenics diehards launched the long-lasting peer-reviewed journal *Mankind Quarterly*. In the coming decades, they published hundreds of papers in this journal. Their continued "scientific" goal: to oppose any scientific basis for civil rights, integrated schools, or interracial marriage. Their *Mankind Quarterly* papers stuffed the footnotes of anti–civil rights legal provisions through the 1960s and '70s.

They proclaimed on the pages of the journal that with the specter of racial admixture and degeneration looming, something drastic had to be done. The future of civilization was at stake.[16]

PART 4

Population Control
(1945–1980)

CHAPTER 14

Puerto Rico: A Surplus Colonial Population

Before World War II, eugenicists moved back and forth between what they called eugenics meetings and population control meetings. This interchange had long-lasting effects. Even though the Holocaust and the Doctors' Trial discredited eugenics in the eyes of many professionals and politicians, even though open financial support from the wealthiest Americans gradually dried up, and even though few spoke anymore of racial "suicide" or "hygiene," old fears of non-whites outreproducing whites didn't disappear after the war. Instead, that older eugenics fear spread—and its solution fell under the banner of population control.

Scratch the surface of the postwar groups championing population control, and you'll find very familiar names: Draper, Ford, DuPont, and Rockefeller. Although fewer channeled their fortunes into intelligence testing and locating white degenerates than they did in the decades before World War II, many of the same donors funded postwar population control interventions in those locations that, just before the war, had been de facto colonies of European and Anglo-American empires. Given their centuries-long situation inside the Anglo-American sphere of influence, Caribbean populations served as some of the easiest targets.

Colonial Eugenics

Clarence Gamble did not need to introduce eugenics to Puerto Rico. It was already there. For much of the 1930s, native Puerto Rican health care workers used the language of eugenics to promote maternal, infant, and child health and welfare. It did not follow the path of Nazi eugenics or even that practiced inside the American Eugenics Triangle. Indeed, the hope of Puerto Rican eugenicists was, as Commissioner of Health Pedro Ortiz put it, to *correct* the bigotry of mainland American health care workers who viewed Puerto Ricans as "an inferior stock, poor, ignorant and degenerated."[1]

But when Clarence Gamble, heir to the Procter & Gamble soap fortune, arrived in the late 1930s, he reappropriated the language of eugenics for his own purposes. Instead of maternal health or children's well-being, Gamble's mission in Puerto Rico would be halting the pernicious slide into degeneration through "population control" via the benevolence of "tropical medicine."

Puerto Ricans long suspected that the health care offered by white American physicians under the heading of tropical medicine had grim strings attached. Gamble made these strings explicit. By taking over and reorganizing the Asociación pro Salud Maternal e Infantil (Maternal and Child Health Association), Gamble pushed spermicides

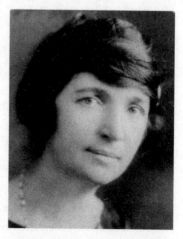

Margaret Sanger, founder of the American Birth Control League

as a means to reduce what he claimed was overpopulation, which led to poverty. He actually thwarted a growing relationship with Margaret Sanger's American Birth Control League (ABCL), which stressed female choice in birth control, in favor of a physician-directed program funded by the Rockefeller Foundation that was predicated on reducing the number of babies born to Puerto Rican women. Gamble also courted pharmaceutical companies. Increasingly, G. D. Searle & Co. and Hoffmann-La Roche, among others, saw the Caribbean as natural laboratories for their products. Gamble promoted his view by publishing medical articles extolling spermicides, based on field trials run in Puerto Rico and Haiti through the 1940s.

The problem was that spermicides didn't work very well. Too many Puerto Rican women who supposedly learned how to use them properly nevertheless became pregnant. Surgical sterilization quickly became a fallback solution for US administrators, who saw the entire island population as far too fecund.

"La Sombra Funesta"—the Sinister Shadow—is what Puerto Ricans called Major General Blanton Winship, a veteran of the Spanish–American War and World War I and President Franklin D. Roosevelt's pick, in 1934, to govern Puerto Rico.[2] From the time the US seized the colonial island from Spain in 1898, American sugar and tobacco corporations bought up most of Puerto Rico's arable land, paying workers pennies and pushing farmers deeper and deeper into poverty. Hurricanes in the autumns of 1936 and 1937 swept away the livelihood of tens of thousands more Puerto Ricans. Unemployment skyrocketed. Labor strikes erupted. A small but frightening student movement threatened violence, adopting

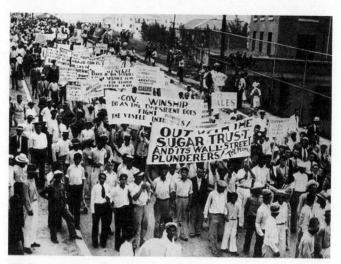

Workers protest Governor Winship and the American sugar corporations.

the black shirts and armbands of Italy's fascists. These Blackshirts mocked the man they called General *Blandón* ("pushover"). But local government insiders suspected that Governor Blanton Winship's job as the first military man to lead Puerto Rico in a generation was not to bring the hope of FDR's New Deal to America's nearest colony but to violently suppress the swelling movement for Puerto Rican independence—just as he had done not long before in the Philippines.[3]

In February 1937, Governor Winship promoted the first abortion and sterilization laws on the island. While, on the one hand, they appeared to offer greater reproductive freedom to Puerto Rican women, that wasn't Winship's intent. He wanted these eugenics measures to "improve the human race"—by decreasing the number of Puerto Ricans.[4]

In 1939, after many accusations of corruption and statesponsored violence against the population, FDR replaced Winship with Rexford Tugwell, one of FDR's original Brain

Trust. Together with Luis Muñoz Marín, the president of the Puerto Rican Senate, Tugwell launched "Operation Bootstrap," a New Deal–esque program intended to industrialize Puerto Rico and reduce unemployment. From the 1930s to the 1960s, Puerto Ricans steadily moved from plantations into the cities for factory jobs. Soon government officials repeated their eugenics message, heard first by Gamble, then by Governor Winship: Puerto Rico was too full of Puerto Ricans. They maintained this claim through the 1940s. They repeated it even though the Puerto Rican birthrate was already lower than that of other Caribbean Islands. They parroted it into the 1950s despite having no hard data showing that overpopulation—rather than exploitation by corporations propped up by the US government—explained Puerto Rican poverty. And, despite protests from the Catholic Church, who saw generations of slavery and racism behind the rhetoric, government officials insisted that "population control" was the solution. Even Governor Muñoz Marín toed the line on this message, despite his otherwise populist reputation. He was too afraid to lose Operation Bootstrap, the American industrial investment attracted by Puerto Rico's low taxes and even lower wages.

> "I rather dislike to think that our falling fertility must be supplemented by these people."
> —Governor Rexford Tugwell[5]

Physicians also echoed those sentiments of Gamble's, Winship's, and Tugwell's—that managing the "surplus population" of Puerto Rico would be the key to health and economic benefits.[6] (Or at least that it would decrease the number of people who might join demonstrations against US colonialism.) According to one survey, some 80 percent of physicians in Puerto Rico favored the female sterilization procedure—*la operación*, as the locals dubbed it.[7] Their support continued through World War II and beyond; even after news emerged of the Nazi weaponization of eugenics to a level never before witnessed; even after the Nuremberg Code (1947) established informed consent of patients. Physicians in mid-century Puerto Rico, and the politicians and nonprofit organizations that interacted with them, saw breeding of the less desirable as a major contributor toward societal degeneration. To tamp down on their reproduction, physicians decided to take matters into their own hands.[8]

After a World War II boost, the economy in Puerto Rico slumped again. Families had too few options. Emigration to Miami and New York City rapidly increased. In the wake of Winfield's laws, surgical sterilizations of women did, too.

Though health care providers supposedly obtained permission to sterilize, consent wasn't actually necessary—the Nuremberg laws formulated after the Nazi Doctors' Trials were not legally binding on Americans. The US possessed no more legally stringent medical code requiring consent, even for white patients, until 1962. Still, historians find little evidence of a coordinated eugenic sterilization campaign on the island: Puerto Rican women did request to be sterilized as a means of controlling their own reproductive health and economic well-being, even though their male partners rarely followed suit.[9]

But these waters are extremely muddy. Women later reported intense pressure by nurses and surgeons for bilateral salpingectomies.[10] A salpingectomy is a surgical procedure to remove one (unilateral) or both (bilateral) fallopian tubes;

the fallopian tubes move eggs into the uterus for conception. In a series of interviews conducted in the 1980s, almost one in five Puerto Rican women confirmed that they had never given explicit consent for sterilization.[11] Mothers already in the hospital to give birth found themselves on the receiving end of *la operación* without fully realizing what had happened. Though we will never know the exact total, interviews suggest a staggering number of surgeries—maybe a third of all Puerto Rican women.[12] Maybe many more. By 1968, a higher percentage of women of childbearing age had been sterilized in Puerto Rico than anywhere else in the world.[13]

Beyond the surgeries themselves, the notion of "surplus population" in Puerto Rico seemed, at least to pharmaceutical companies, an ethical license to test new contraceptives and abortifacients. G. D. Searle & Co. went first.

> "[We need] a cage of ovulating females to experiment with."
> —Katherine McCormick, a major funder of the birth control pill trials, to Margaret Sanger, 1955[14]

By 1952, John Rock, a gynecologist, and Gregory Pincus, a biochemist, both associated with Harvard University, became convinced that hormones held the key to contraception. Rock had already tried using progesterone as a high-dosage infertility treatment on his low-income patients at the Free Hospital for Women in the town of Brookline, part of the Boston metropolitan area. Around 15 percent of his patients became pregnant through what was called the "Rock rebound." Paradoxically, Pincus used the same hormone to *prevent* pregnancy in rabbits. After meeting up at a conference, Rock and Pincus decided to launch a more concerted trial on sixty patients at the Free Hospital for Women to determine the effect of progesterone on the menstrual cycle. Half of the women disliked the side effects and quit. But this didn't deter Rock and Pincus; they saw real potential, and not just for fame and fortune. As Rock flatly stated in a radio interview years later, "People like to have babies, and this is particularly so among primitive peoples."[15] Their work could be the magic bullet so many had been looking for—a legal way to control non-white reproduction.

And there were even louder echoes of eugenics past. After testing progesterone pills on mentally ill women at the Worcester State Hospital in 1954, Pincus then cut them open to check ovulation. A year later, he devised a set of experiments on the genitals of mentally ill men to test their "castration anxiety." Even sympathetic reviewers of Pincus's work expressed concerns that he was treating patients like "guinea pigs." Old rumors resurfaced that he was not granted tenure at Harvard University back in 1937 due to questionable experiments. But by 1955, Pincus could shrug all that off. He had more funding than ever, through a wealthy comrade of Margaret Sanger, who was also a major funder of Worcester State Hospital, and a believer in the power of hormones: Katherine D. McCormick. To test their pills, McCormick believed Rock and Pincus would need a "'cage' of ovulating females to experiment with."[16] They found their cage in the Rio Piedras neighborhood of San Juan, Puerto Rico, a housing development for agricultural laborers who had left their farms because of Operation Bootstrap.

There are two versions of what happened next. In the tale told and retold in the continental US over the next

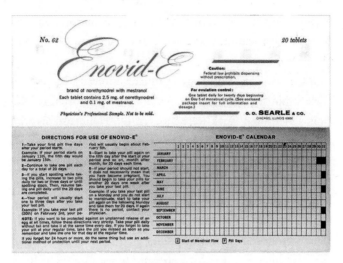

Enovid package, 1960s

half century, "the pill" was produced from a combination of McCormick's money, Sanger's inspiration, Rock's connections, and Pincus's persistence and ingenuity—not to mention the fortuitous discovery by a biochemistry team in Mexico led by Carl Djerassi that common yams were a renewable source of hormones similar to progesterone. Beginning in 1956, hundreds of women in San Juan overwhelmingly demonstrated that the pill made by Searle & Co. and sold under the brand name Enovid prevented pregnancy. With a shrinking birthrate, the standard of living in Puerto Rico increased.[17] On the mainland, the Food and Drug Administration (FDA) saw the light and approved "the pill" for female contraception in 1960. Large numbers of women, for the first time in human history, could free themselves from the oppression of unwanted motherhood. And millions of middle- and upper-class American women did just that. In *Griswold v. Connecticut* (1965) and *Eisenstadt v. Baird* (1972), the US Supreme Court removed legal barriers to contraception. A sexual revolution followed. Second-wave feminism followed. The remaking of Western culture followed.[18]

In the alternative version, penned, ironically, by second-wave feminist scholars in the wake of this purported revolution, Pincus and Rock were modern Dr. Frankensteins who treated Puerto Rican women as lab rats for their experiments and ignored warning signs that their drugs caused serious side effects. Physicians administering Enovid reported blood clots, occasionally leading to more serious complications, including death. The FDA had hesitated to grant their approval until Pincus produced additional results, after shifting the locus of the experiments to rural patients in Humacao, Puerto Rico, and Port-au-Prince, Haiti—looking for that perfect "cage."[19] The Catholic Church pushed back at every juncture, elevating opposition to chemical and surgical birth control to a doctrinal priority. Pope Paul VI's *Humanae Vitae* (1968) denounced state-sponsored sterilization campaigns and warned that widespread contraception would make it easier for men to view women merely as a means of sexual gratification.[20] Yet the capitalist incentive promoted by American industries that had taken advantage of Operation Bootstrap, and American imperialism more broadly, toppled sentimental religious barriers. Puerto Rican women couldn't resist falling into the Western pharmaceutical machine, runs this narrative.

More recent scholars find some truth on both sides. Yet, they emphasize that, crucially, both accounts deny agency to Puerto Rican women. Whatever Rock, Pincus, and other male physicians intended, working-class women made conscious choices to experience the liberation of birth control. Savvy female health care providers informed and assisted them.

Persistent feminists pushed for the liberation of oral contraceptives. All were agents of their own destinies, pioneers breaking through centuries of general prejudice against allowing women to have that control and actual laws—Anthony Comstock's Laws, first deployed against Victoria Woodhull's followers generations earlier—and against contraception specifically.[21] To suggest otherwise is to fall into the same colonial mindset: well-intentioned but infantilizing and, therefore, still sexist and racist.[22]

The official eugenics movement in Puerto Rico claimed to have sterilized fewer than one hundred mentally ill patients over three decades. With such a small number of these sorts of sterilizations, and with the explicit wish of many working-class women in Puerto Rico to receive contraception, how could the story of Puerto Rico be a part of this larger eugenics story?

Here's how: After World War II, the rhetoric surrounding eugenics changed. "Eugenics" became a word associated with Nazis. But the impulse continued for those with wealth and status to reduce the reproductive capabilities of those without it, along with the justification that this halted degeneration or overpopulation or "entrenched poverty." White physicians, scientists, and philanthropists interested in controlling brown bodies initiated the studies of, sought funding for, and promoted the pill using the language of population control on "surplus" non-whites. Catholic leaders in Puerto Rico charged American imperialism. African American leaders feared that the wide distribution of the pill by white physicians signaled out-and-out genocide of non-whites. Given the long history of powerful whites manipulating the reproduction of less powerful non-whites, it seems hazardous to swat away these concerns so easily.

At minimum, we should acknowledge the steady stream of complaints—even after oral contraceptive trials ended in the mid-1960s—by Puerto Rican mothers about surgeons who continued to administer "la operación" without clear consent. Surgical sterilization remained at a high rate in Puerto Rico, even as white women experienced the sexual revolution brought on by the pill.[23] Population control to relieve poor, overcrowded Puerto Rico haunted the island even as economic conditions improved, even after eugenics was no longer discussed.

Ironically, the contraceptive Enovid itself was too expensive, hanging just out of reach for the very women who acted as Pincus and Rock's test subjects. By then, the doctors had flown back to Massachusetts, now famous as the men who granted freedom to women, medical saviors who released mothers from the shackles of primitive traditions and too many children.[24]

CHAPTER 15

The Population Control
Industrial Complex

The US government put its official stamp of approval on population control almost as soon as the Cold War began. And, whatever their rhetoric, international population control—as promoted by powerful governmental, non-governmental, and corporate organizations during the 1950s through '70s—had little to do with empowering the poor in Latin America, the Caribbean, or Southeast Asia to take control of their own bodies and families. Just as they expressed in international congresses held before World War II, advocates for population control most often advocated controlling the fertility of non-white women to solve social problems. From time to time, they explicitly advocated anti-immigration policies. To be sure, their feel-good corporate marketing might say otherwise, yet even in the wake of Nazi atrocities, European and American population control organizations never discarded the core eugenics assumption: that they could properly weigh which pregnancies were "wanted"—and which were not.[1]

In 1949, John D. Rockefeller III, heir to the Standard Oil fortune, heard a rumor from two fellow trustees of the Rockefeller Foundation, John Foster Dulles and Dean Rusk—political pugilists with outsized influences on American foreign policy throughout several presidential administrations.

Agents sent by the Truman administration to learn why China turned communist had returned from East Asia with a detailed report. But John III, known for traveling widely in Asia, believed he already knew why: too many peasants. Promises of a revolution by the proletariat would inevitably lure those with too many mouths to feed and too few resources, even if the leaders of that revolution were the bloodthirsty Mao or Stalin.

Spurred by his conversation with Dulles and Rusk, John III quickly assembled a group of social scientists, government officials, and business tycoons. He called the group the Population Council. Their mission would be to convince the wealthy and powerful around the world that "the relationship of population to material and cultural resources of the world represents one of the most crucial and urgent problems of the day."[2] Rockefeller wouldn't pressure his magnates to redistribute much of *their own* great power or wealth. If capitalists in

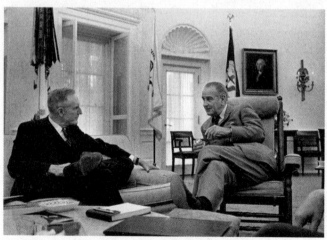

John D. Rockefeller III meeting with President Lyndon B. Johnson in the Oval Office, 1968

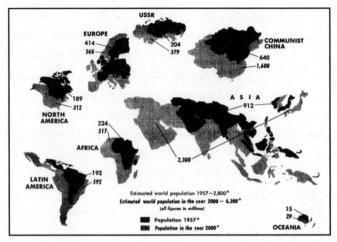

President Eisenhower tasked the Draper Committee to review military assistance to combat the spread of communism. Though unrelated to military projects, reducing birthrates in "third world" nations emerged as a top concern for the Committee.

the US and Europe wanted to contain communism, it would be much better, he intimated, to practice Cold War containment on all the poor non-whites who were bringing too many babies into the world in the first place.

By the mid-1950s, the Population Council had embedded itself deeply enough in the military-industrial complex to convince generals. They prodded the president and retired five-star general, Dwight D. Eisenhower, who, in 1958, launched the President's Committee to Study the US Military Assistance Program, better known as the Draper Committee, with former Under Secretary of War, Major General William H. Draper Jr., as its head. General Draper gathered a ten-man circle of bankers, military brass, and CEOs, including James E. Webb (the telescope's namesake, who left the petroleum industry to join the Draper Committee en route to directing JFK's NASA moon shot).

The Draper Committee foregrounded the birth rate of so-called Third World nations, Puerto Rico included, as a pressing issue for US foreign policy.[3] Their reporting convinced Eisenhower of a population problem in the roughly one-third of the world that had not yet subscribed to American capitalism or Soviet communism (i.e., the "Third World"). Overpopulation, they warned Ike, would inexorably lead these mostly poor countries into the arms of the Soviet/Chinese menace. It was exactly what Lothrop Stoddard predicted in *The Revolt Against Civilization* (1922).

The Draper Committee insisted that the US government work with underdeveloped countries to lower their reproduction as a means to contain that communist impulse. And despite the fact that Eisenhower swore his administration would never support "birth control," he publicly announced in a pivotal press conference in December 1959 that the US would attach "population control" as a condition of international aid. He then departed for his eleven-country "mission of peace and goodwill" to some of the very countries targeted.[4]

At first, Ike remained detached from the means of this conditional provision. *It wasn't America's job to police the birth rates of other nations*, he thought. But that sentiment gradually changed after he left the presidency in 1961. The Lyndon B. Johnson administration convinced him. That's primarily because LBJ's allies pushed Congress repeatedly to increase aid and anti-poverty programs both domestically and internationally. Republicans, including Eisenhower, objected. American wealth should not go to non-white countries without strings of population control attached. Southern Democrats agreed. So, ironically, the population control message from Eisenhower, a Republican, found the greatest purchase in the

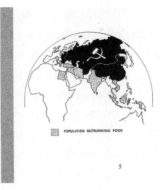

This 1950s Planned Parenthood pamphlet stressed population control as a Cold War necessity to combat the spread of communism.

Senate Government Operations subcommittee, led by Southern Democrats.[5]

Though Eisenhower and the 1960s successor organization to his Draper Committee (more on them below) ostensibly directed their rhetoric at controlling reproduction in foreign populations, they also stressed a domestic application of population control. This sounded all too familiar to those with knowledge of the American eugenics movement. Perhaps that's because, behind the scenes, *another* Draper was at work.

Wickliffe Preston Draper (not a direct relative of General William H. Draper Jr.) had long been channeling the family fortune from textile manufacturing into the eugenics movement. Convinced that race mixing was degenerating society, Wickliffe Draper spent a considerable amount of his own money funding research that emphasized the same old biological hierarchies supposedly discovered in the nineteenth century. Social scientists funded by Wickliffe Draper built up support for IQ, not skull size, as a real measure of racial difference.

Draper helped fund Laughlin's US tour of the Nazi-produced films *Das Erbe* (1935) and *Erbkrank* (1936). Then, after

World War II, as the civil rights movement gained momentum, Draper's foundation—the Pioneer Fund—opened the financial spigot to pro-segregationists for multiple generations. Draper money funded the biologist Wesley Critz George and the psychologist Audrey Shuey, who fought the US Supreme Court's decision in *Brown v. Board of Education of Topeka, Kansas* (1954)—the case that racially integrated American schools. Draper money also backed the psychologist Arthur Jensen, who published research in the *Harvard Educational Review* that supposedly found rock-solid evidence for racial intelligence differences.[6] Draper money propped up William Shockley, who, in the 1960s and beyond, advocated for the reestablishment of laws permitting eugenic sterilization of non-whites. Draper money even flowed to the former fascist Henry Garrett, chair of Columbia University's psychology department, who used the funds to launch *Mankind Quarterly*, a peer-reviewed academic journal (mentioned in the previous chapter) that promoted new research into those old canards of societal degeneration through race mixing and overpopulation by non-whites.[7] On issue after issue, the only solutions offered, unsurprisingly, were segregation and sterilization. Both at home

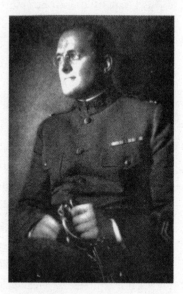

Wickliffe P. Draper, founder of the anti-immigration and pro–racial segregation Pioneer Fund.

and abroad, the unfit were having too many babies. Former Nazi doctors like Otmar von Verschuer found a publication home in *Mankind Quarterly*.

Through separate pursuits, both the overtly bigoted Wickliffe Draper and the more pragmatic General William H. Draper combined to frighten even dedicated humanitarians like Eisenhower. In June 1965, Ike wrote an urgent letter to *The New York Times*.

> I must refer to reported instances . . . of the repetitive production of children by unwed mothers, apparently lured by the resulting increase in income from welfare funds. . . . When this is repeated to the point of habit, society will find itself in the curious position of spending money with one hand to slow up population growth among responsible families and with the other providing financial incentive for increased production by the ignorant, feeble-minded, or lazy. . . . If research should uncover no effective measures other than legal sterilization, a final resort to this method unquestionably would shock great segments of our citizenry.[8]

The need to return to involuntary sterilization could not be ruled out entirely inside the US, Eisenhower implied. And that went double for other countries. It's unclear whether Ike was simply ignorant of the fact that "research" had already developed effective oral contraceptives or that he truly believed "legal sterilization" had to remain on the table because, as Clarence Gamble believed of Puerto Rico, poor women could not be trusted to use contraceptives effectively.[9]

By the mid-1960s, General W. H. Draper (*note*: not Wickliffe Draper) had moved out of cloistered government committees and into the public forum. He founded the Population Crisis Committee (PCC) alongside two industrial potentates: Lammot du Pont Copeland, inheritor of the DuPont chemical fortune (the du Pont Copelands funded eugenics congresses in the 1920s), and Hugh Everett Moore, the founder and president of the Dixie Cup company. Moore had already published the booklet *The Population Bomb Is Everyone's Baby* in 1954—the model for the more widely known *Population Bomb* written by Paul Ehrlich a decade later, as we'll soon encounter.[10]

Through the intense lobbying of Draper, du Pont Copeland, and Moore, the PCC pushed the US Agency for International Development (USAID) to support population control in some of the very countries Eisenhower visited during his goodwill tour back in 1959. And through USAID, even the United Nations would get behind the population control project. In Vietnam, for instance, USAID and the PCC foisted birth control pharmaceuticals on the local populace to combat communism, blaming Southeast Asian poverty not on French colonialist policies, corrupt Western-backed Vietnamese leaders, or American napalm being dropped on agricultural fields, but on ignorant mothers.[11]

Throughout the mid-century period of intense American military and CIA-led interventions in East Asia, the Near East, the Caribbean, and Latin America, American government agents and non-governmental organizations (NGOs) constructed the population control industrial complex. Health care workers from North Africa to Taiwan saw their pay tied to the number of intrauterine devices (IUDs) they inserted into women, with or without consent. In the Philippines, American aid workers reportedly delivered birth control pills by tossing them from helicopters. Across the "Third World," physicians sterilized thousands, often coercively, sometimes illegally, and frequently under unsafe conditions. Scholarships, grants to conferences, awards, and favorable publicity encouraged social and economic elites from the targeted populations to join with the US- , UK- , and EU-led population control initiatives and agencies. Alongside USAID, the World Bank and the UN Fund for Population Activities pressured governments to design and implement their own population control policies.[12]

It's important to point out that overt expressions of malice did not accompany these initiatives—because it's too easy when reading the above to imagine a *Dr. Strangelove*–esque cabal of men arguing in a smoke-filled underground war room, deriving ways to persecute some target population. Eugenics never worked that way. Policymakers (those already in power) believed they were doing what was in their own best interests by attempting to reduce the ability of the politically almost powerless poor to add more children to their families, lest the world be overrun by too many of the wrong sorts.

> "The single greatest failure of foresight—at all levels of government—over the past generation has been in areas connected with expanding population. Government and legislatures have frequently failed to appreciate the demands which continued population growth would impose on the public sector."
> —President Richard M. Nixon, July 18, 1969[13]

Instead, we should envision eugenics in mid-century in a constant three-sided tension. On one side, powerful Western—especially American—forces enacted policy agendas to serve (at least explicitly) Cold War geopolitical ends, with non-white populations, usually mothers, as the target. On another side, women sought greater control over their own reproduction and families; even when fully aware of the population control ideology motivating contraception, abortion, and sterilization measures, women took advantage of the freedom offered or resisted the tools that restricted them. And a third side, often caught between these other two, was when well-intentioned health care workers advocated both for patients and for their own authority to deliver care in their own ways. Increasingly, a fourth factor entered the conversation and put additional pressure on governments, mothers, and health care providers alike: the pharmaceutical companies that marketed contraceptives.

Even in medical scenarios where controlling the reproduction of non-white populations was announced as an overt pursuit, physicians and nurses, indigenous or from Western countries themselves, rendered care that poor patients simply wouldn't have had otherwise. Health officials in Puerto Rico, Latin America, and Southeast Asia weren't dupes.[14] Yet, they weren't entirely able to extricate themselves, or their patients, from the external pressure to bring fewer non-white babies into the world.

CHAPTER 16

The Population Bomb Bomb

It's not hard to understand why, even when assisted by sympathetic health care workers, mothers in the 1960s in nations very recently considered colonies by Europeans (for example, Puerto Rico, most of Africa, Southeast Asia, much of South America) found it difficult to push back against the notion of population control. Introduction of the pill and other pharmaceutical birth control interventions amplified the private and non-governmental efforts to control the population of non-whites around the world in tandem with governmental ones. Academics joined the fray as well. The fears of eugenicists past reappeared in seemingly environmentally conscious books such as Frederick Osborn's *Our Plundered Planet* (1948). You might recall this Osborn's famous uncle, H. F. Osborn, friends with Madison Grant and autocratic leader of the American Museum of Natural History, plus host to two international eugenics congresses. The postwar environmental movement retained many connections with the pre-1930s eugenics movement.[1]

The weeds of eugenics sentiments sprouted once again in the 1960s work of Melvin Ketchel, a physiologist at Tufts University School of Medicine; Garrett Hardin, a biologist at the University of California, Santa Barbara; and Paul Ehrlich, a butterfly specialist at Stanford University. Infamously, they feared overpopulation so much that they floated the idea of dumping contraceptives into drinking water in Asia and Africa.[2] Anything less than Zero Population Growth (ZPG), a movement Ehrlich founded in 1968—rebranded in 2002 as Population Connection—spelled disaster for the whole planet.[3]

Ehrlich borrowed the title of his bestselling *The Population Bomb* (1968) directly from works circulating among General W. H. Draper Jr.'s Population Crisis Committee a decade earlier.[4] The themes

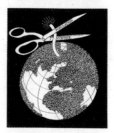

THE POPULATION BOMB THREATENS THE PEACE OF THE WORLD

SO WHAT ARE WE DOING ABOUT IT?

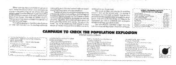

The notion of population as a bomb began in the 1950s and resonated through the last half of the twentieth century. To some scientists, Zero Population Growth (ZPG) appeared to be the best answer.

Ehrlich channeled can be found in scores of previously published materials, from Stoddard's *The Rising Tide of Color* (1920) onward. But Ehrlich did explicitly disassociate himself with earlier scientific racism. Ehrlich's *Population Bomb* made so much more of an impression on the minds of American and Europeans than any of these other writings because of its apocalyptic rhetoric—you'd need to go back to Joseph Arthur de Gobineau to find its equivalent. "The battle to feed all of humanity is over," Ehrlich pronounced.

> "In the 1970s the world will undergo famines—hundreds of millions of people are going to starve to death in spite of any crash programs embarked upon now. At this late date nothing can prevent a substantial increase in the world death rate."
>
> —Paul Ehrlich[5]

Back in the nineteenth century, one of the major fears was that in a world of limited resources, the profligate degenerates, who could not or would not manage their family size, would drive the planet into a population "trap" even if superior people had fewer children. That worry bubbled to the surface again in Ehrlich's *Population Bomb*, now in the guise of Earth-friendly environmentalism. Garrett Hardin's pseudo-history, "The Tragedy of the Commons," appeared in *Science* at the same time, suggesting that the fears were well founded: Humanity had blithely waltzed into Malthusian traps in the past and, unless Western countries intervened in the Third World, a cataclysmic problem was around the corner.

Defusing the Bomb

Ehrlich strongly criticized the petroleum industry, and he didn't spare Western consumers, either: Each white person consumed many times more

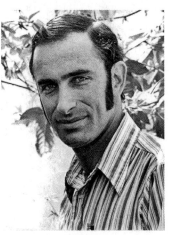

Paul Ehrlich in 1974

than their fair share. Corporations pulled too many resources out of the earth, creating shiny baubles for Westerners who already had plenty. In developed countries, pollution generated by industries making those novelties threatened to render the environment too warm, via the greenhouse effect (yes, projected in 1968), and too toxic for the agriculture needed to sustain several billion additional humans. "There will never be 7 billion people by the year 2000," Ehrlich predicted in 1970, when there were 3.7 billion people.

But those were general criticisms of corporations and consumers. Ehrlich saved his actual *policy* recommendations for the "cancer of population growth."[6] "Undeveloped" countries fed this cancer. The populations of Kenya, Nigeria, Turkey, Indonesia, the Philippines, Brazil, Costa Rica, and El Salvador were on track to double by the 1980s or '90s, he said. And look at India, which he visited in 1966. South Central Asia already spilled over with too many mouths to feed. The only question, he surmised, was whether global population would halt below seven billion, because of Malthusian tragedies like "famine, plague, or war," or because governments intelligently scripted and enforced population control policies to avoid these three.[7] (Spoiler alert: The world is currently feeding more than Ehrlich's projections.)

> "A feud about how to deal with overpopulation surfaced in Stockholm, between Ehrlich and his nemesis, Barry Commoner, whose popular book *The Closing Circle* (1971) directly criticized Ehrlich's population-bomb thesis. . . . Commoner's argument was that population policies weren't needed because what was called 'the demographic transition' would

take care of everything—all you had to do was help
poor people get less poor, and they would have fewer
children. Ehrlich insisted that the situation was way
too serious for that approach, and it wouldn't work
anyway: You needed harsh government programs to
drive down the birthrate."

—Stewart Brand, environmental activist (2010)[8]

After spinning several nightmare scenarios, Ehrlich proposed his *best* case: that by the mid-1970s, the US would dra-
conianly withdraw food subsidies, and much of Asia, Africa,
South America, and the Near East would descend into riots
and civil war, killing millions. Pro-Soviet governments would
collapse. An enlightened pope would encourage his Span-
ish-speaking flock to seek abortions and practice contraception. Eventually, pro-American nations and the UN Security
Council (minus the USSR and China, which by then would
have ceased to exist) would orchestrate "area rehabilitation,"
including marriage and child restrictions throughout much
of the undeveloped world. By 1985, Ehrlich hoped, fears of a
Black and Brown planet could be snuffed out.

Ehrlich had ideas for how non-white population control
could be accomplished. But, like Clarence Gamble in Puerto
Rico, Ehrlich scoffed at doing it through "family planning."
John D. Rockefeller III's old Population Council had settled
on that method, which mostly meant education and distributing intrauterine devices (IUDs) in poor countries. But could
you trust poor mothers to have the *correct* number of children? He, Hardin, and others of their ilk preferred "population policy." "Soft" population policy meant the West would

instruct societies on how many children they actually *needed* and would create "disincentives" through changing taxes, school systems, and social norms. "Hard" population policy, though, was probably required: stringently enforced laws limiting the number of children to two or fewer.[9]

Western journalists, academics, entertainers, and policymakers trumpeted *The Population Bomb* and the Zero Population Growth (ZPG) movement it birthed as ecologically imperative. Americans were "Squeezing into the '70s," declared *Life* magazine. Even Disney got into the act. Donald Duck illustrated family planning in a public service cartoon using a Mexican father of three as a central protagonist who concedes to the narrator's wishes that they try pills and devices to establish a new "balance" between births and deaths.[10] Ehrlich himself became a regular guest on *The Tonight Show Starring Johnny Carson* on NBC. After Ehrlich's first appearance, Carson recalled seeing the highest audience engagement of any guest. Though none of his predictions from *The Population Bomb* came to pass, Ehrlich had great stage presence for a scientist and gave voice to deeply held fears of a society on the threshold of disaster. Into the 1980s, Ehrlich used Carson's show to speak directly to millions of Americans about their "declining quality of life" in the face of environmental degradation, the threat of nuclear war, and illegal Mexican immigration.[11]

"Smog covers the earth. The oxygen is depleted. Love is encouraged. But the penalty for birth is death. THE TIME IS TOMORROW AND THERE'S NO TIME LEFT."
—from a promotional poster for the film *Z. P. G.* (1972) inspired by Ehrlich's *The Population Bomb*

Outside the US, however, attempts to control the population of non-whites encountered significant opposition. This came to a head at the World Population Conference held in Bucharest, Romania, in 1974. Organizers intended the conference to be a celebration of Western population control efforts, highlighting IUDs, the pill, and other contraceptive methods. Meeting planners expected to ratify a "World Population Plan of Action." Instead, countries across the globe dug in their heels, slamming the population control establishment backed by the US, the UK, and the EU as only superficially humanitarian.[12] The Vatican spoke up against America's profound blindness toward its own history of abusing the weakest, and the way in which that history blindness twisted any attempt at population control. Also, it turned out, the ZPG's statistics didn't hold up.

Nevertheless, at least in the so-called First World in the last quarter of the twentieth century, the population control movement inspired by *The Population Bomb* continued to

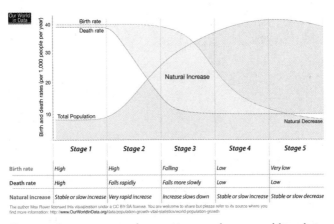

	Stage 1	Stage 2	Stage 3	Stage 4	Stage 5
Birth rate	High	High	Falling	Low	Very low
Death rate	High	Falls rapidly	Falls more slowly	Low	Low
Natural increase	Stable or slow increase	Very rapid increase	Increase slows down	Stable or slow increase	Stable or slow decrease

Demographers now suggest that as nation-states become wealthier, their populations transition from high birth and death rates to lower birth and death rates, slowing and even reversing population growth.[13]

hold together seemingly opposed groups: feminists, who earnestly wanted to extend education and reproductive rights to marginalized women; environmentalists, who earnestly wanted to conserve natural resources and living things as they currently existed on Earth; and those powerful few who earnestly believed the future of the planet should not be left up to the undeserving.[14] As one policy analyst put it, "Today population control—a philosophy that subordinates people's need for control over their own bodies and lives to dubious economic and political imperatives—knows no borders."[15]

CHAPTER 17

Emergencies

It was late, and Delhi remained soupy, above 100 degrees. Paul Ehrlich and his tired family crawled through the smelly, loud, crowded streets in a dilapidated taxi, longing for their hotel. You can hear the disgust in Ehrlich's recounting: "People eating, people washing, people sleeping. People visiting, arguing and screaming. People thrusting their hands through the taxi window, begging. People defecating and urinating. People clinging to buses. People herding animals."[1] A world incomprehensible, compared to their upper-middle-class life in California. In 1965, President Lyndon B. Johnson called global population growth one of the major concerns of the age. "Let us act on the fact that less than five dollars invested in population control," LBJ intoned to the UN, "is worth a hundred dollars invested in economic growth."[2] Juxtaposed with his experience baking in Delhi in 1966, that message turned Ehrlich toward population control as promoted by Draper's Population Crisis Committee. Ehrlich also read the apocalyptic book *Famine 1975! America's Decision: Who Will Survive?* (1967), predicting mass famines in India within the next decade—which served as a further justification. Together, these experiences set him on the path to the *Population Bomb* project. Ehrlich conveniently ignored that Paris, France, which he enjoyed, contained almost triple the population of Delhi at the time he visited.[3]

Unbeknownst to Ehrlich, NGOs and influential members of both the US government and the United Nations were paying attention. Language of race suicide and eugenic sterilization had faded into the background. The Cold War political-military incentive for population control to halt the "domino effect" of poor countries converting to communism likewise slowly gave way. Yet the propensity for predominantly white America to influence the reproduction of predominantly non-white populations continued to intensify, though now under humanitarian and environmentalist initiatives. Ripples of population control strategies, themselves derived from eugenics, continue today.

Since the 1950s, the Ford Foundation, the wealthiest philanthropic organization on the planet, had been pushing hard for population control in India. Dr. Sushila Nayar, the late Mahatma Gandhi's influential physician, disapproved of artificial contraceptives promoted by Western corporations, and much of the Indian government agreed with her. Still, Ford Foundation officials successfully smuggled in the double-S Lippes loops IUDs as Christmas-tree ornaments. By 1966, doctors had inserted them into over one million Indian women.[4] Indian health ministers and physicians grew suspicious of the motivations behind such schemes and resisted foreign-funded "family planning" NGOs. The US government, however, was about to put its thumb on the scale.

Prime Minister Indira Gandhi came to Washington in March 1966 to request greater food aid. Secretary of State Dean Rusk (who over a decade earlier had encouraged John D. Rockefeller III to set up his Population Council) and President Johnson agreed to the aid. In exchange, they demanded a "massive effort" from Gandhi on population control. True to her word, Gandhi's government set IUD insertion and sterilization quotas, paying provinces and physicians the equivalent of one to three days' wages per IUD inserted and up to two weeks' wages for a surgical sterilization.[5] But these incentives proved too slow from the West's perspective, given the dire predictions being made by Ehrlich and ZPG, among others.

On March 16, 1970, President Nixon created the Commission on Population Growth and the American Future (CPGAF) based on the recommendations of Secretary of State Henry Kissinger, who had followed Ehrlich's predictions and the work of American NGOs pushing for population control in India. Nixon assigned John III, now in his third decade of population control advocacy, to chair the twenty-four-member task force. The CPGAF targeted thirteen countries, placing India at the top of the list.[6]

> "In the brief history of the nation, we have always assumed that progress and the 'good life' are connected with population growth. . . . If that were ever the case, it is not now. . . . We have concluded that no substantial benefits would result from continued growth of the nation's population."
> —The Commission on Population Growth and the American Future (1972)[7]

Four years later, in December 1974, National Security Study Memorandum 200 (NSSM 200), better known as the Kissinger Report, appeared on the desk of the newly sworn-in president, Gerald Ford. Since the Eisenhower administration, conservatives and liberals alike had insisted that foreign aid to less developed countries (LDCs) should be conditional upon population control measures. By the mid-1970s, this usually meant the wide distribution of the pill, IUDs, and condoms. Yet, as another Nixon holdover, Dr. Reimert Ravenholt at the US Agency for International Development (USAID) stressed, to save the degenerating world it might be necessary to sterilize a quarter of its women—voluntarily, of course.[8] With Kissinger at the helm and NSSM 200 as the guiding principle, the Ford administration already appeared poised to take "hard" population policy very seriously.[9]

Then came "The Emergency."

Beset by internal conflict and external pressures, in 1975, Prime Minister Gandhi suspended civil liberties and promised to use her new dictatorial powers to eliminate poverty. She did so by working to eradicate the poor. Under the direction of her son, Sanjay, the Indian government instituted policies that restricted food and medical care and even withheld paychecks unless those targeted received sterilizations. They pressured schools to expel students if their parents refused to be sterilized. From small provinces to large cities, police and government officials rounded up men for vasectomies, often in mobile units that scoured fields at night looking for those who fled their homes to hide. "All they wanted were men. Any man," Khandu Genu Kamble, a sterilized sanitation worker, later recalled. "We didn't complain because the [government] warned us that we'd lose our jobs if we did."[10] Between six and eight million men and women underwent sterilization in the latter half of 1976 alone, dwarfing US sterilizations and even the Nazi-instigated campaign in the 1930s.[11] Rounded-up patients filled schools, clubs, and government buildings. Physicians sterilized patients in assembly line fashion. "Some doctors performed the surgery in minutes," admitted Dr.

Arvind Bhopalkar, a physician who was conscripted into sterilization surgeries during The Emergency, "others took hours and struggled. It was medically unethical."[12] Thousands of the sterilized died from infection. Thousands more died in the crackdown against the riots protesting these policies.

The US reacted with cautious optimism. The Ford White House urged officials "to refrain from public comment on forced-paced measures" by Gandhi's government.[13] When he learned of it, Robert S. McNamara, the head of the World Bank and formerly the architect of the Vietnam War, glowed: "At long last, India is moving to effectively address its population problem."[14]

Gandhi's "Emergency" lasted only two years—her government lost in a landslide in 1977. Still, more than ten million people went under the knife. And that legacy of coerced surgical sterilization for the poor in India continues sporadically through the present, often resulting in physician error and patient death. In reaction, men now avoid contraception

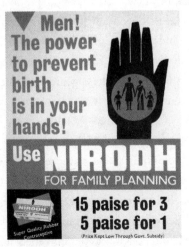

A 1960s Indian family planning poster

altogether.[15] For decades, the sterilized have been largely women, and, until India's high court banned the practice in 2016, the surgeries often took place in medical camps constructed exclusively for that purpose.[16]

China

The Population Bomb bomb exploded again at the 1979 population conference in Chengdu, China. Based on computer models translated

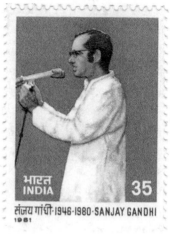

Sanjay Gandhi, who spearheaded India's family planning initiative during the Emergency, pictured here on an Indian postage stamp

from the 1972 jeremiad *Limits to Growth*, Chinese engineers speculated that the country needed to cut its population in half or risk catastrophe. (*Limits to Growth* was produced by the Club of Rome, an exclusive economic forecasting group co-founded by two Italian industrialists and David Rockefeller, brother of John III. Recall that the father of both Rockefeller brothers was one of the key financiers of the eugenics movement in the first half of the century.) Some professional social scientists regarded these models as far too flimsy—"Malthus with a computer."[17] And as insiders reminded the government, the "Late, Long, and Few" Chinese family planning movement of the 1970s had already successfully reduced population growth by half in less than a decade. But the engineers prevailed in persuading Premier Deng Xiaoping and the Chinese Central Committee. China's "One Child Policy" was put into effect in 1980.[18]

For over three decades, China's National Health and Family Planning Commission fined parents who chose to have more than one child. If teachers and other government workers were discovered to have secretly had a second child, they could lose their jobs. Government ministers claimed the policy dropped the projected population of China by four hundred million and prevented famines.[19] Yet almost immediately, credible stories also emerged about coerced contraception and involuntary abortions, sterilizations, and infanticides. Rumors circulated that authorities were reverting to torture to keep parents in line.[20] As a direct result, parents allowed more male than female babies to live, massively skewing sex ratios for many years, the long-term implications of which are only now coming to light.[21]

In 1993, the Public Health Minister proposed a law called "On Eugenics and Health Protection" that required couples with a history of mental illness or venereal disease to take "long-term contraceptive measures," including mandatory abortions and sterilization. After the international community

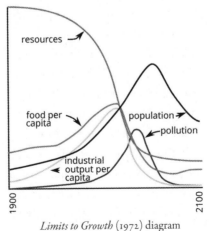

Limits to Growth (1972) diagram

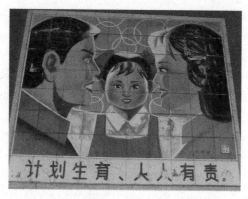

计划生育、人人有责。

One-child policy poster, Shenyang, Liaoning Province, China, c. 1984

erupted in protest at the suggestion, they retitled the bill the "Natal and Health Care Law." In a carefully worded press release, the Public Health Ministry complained that the West had mistakenly attributed Nazi motivations to the new law, which was simply about health care.[22] Even though by the mid-1980s it had become apparent that these policies proved *too* effective, crackdowns continued well into the 2000s, until demographers warned that, ironically, China would soon face the opposite demographic crisis: an aging workforce and too few younger families.

The National People's Congress allowed a two-child policy beginning in 2016, with a third child allowed in rural areas. Still, old eugenic tendencies continued. In the western Xinjiang province, at the same moment that they relaxed the one-child policy on the Han, the ethnic majority, the government began to subject the minority Uyghurs to abortions, IUD insertions, fines, and detentions for having too many children. In Xinjiang, sterilizations climbed from 14 per 100,000 in 2014 to a shocking 250 per 100,000 in 2018, while declining in China overall.[23] Unsurprisingly, this larger campaign has resulted in a Uyghur birth rate crash. International organizations declare it a coordinated genocidal campaign.[24]

Peru

In September 1995, President Alberto Fujimori of Peru appeared at the UN's Fourth World Conference on Women in Beijing. He was the only male head of state to speak there—a celebrated occurrence at the time—and he reiterated that women had the right to control their own fertility. At the very same moment, however, Fujimori's government was instituting a population control strategy targeting indigenous women.[25]

Between 1996 and 1998, the human rights attorney Giulia Tamayo and the Comité de América Latina y el Caribe para la Defensa de los Derechos Humanos de la Mujer (CLADEM; "Latin American and Caribbean Committee for the Defense of Women's Rights") confirmed over 240 allegations of forced contraception and sterilizations leading to at least one death by sepsis. Nearly all of the sterilized were ethnic minority (for example, Quechua) women. But CLADEM suspected this was only the tip of the iceberg: Language barriers, cultural shame, and remote locations proved formidable to voluntary investigators living under Fujimori's autocratic rule.[26] After constructing a telephone-based testimony project, a network of lawyers, human rights activists, and journalists uncovered the sterilization of nearly 272,000 women and 22,000 men.[27] Some reported being tied down and blindfolded by health care workers. Others were threatened with imprisonment of family members if they did not consent. Still others agreed to receive malaria medication only to learn later they were really being given anesthesia and sterilized while unconscious.[28]

Fujimori resigned in 2000 over unrelated corruption charges. In 2009, the Peruvian high court convicted him of human rights violations (again, not related to these sterilizations) and sentenced him to twenty-five years in prison. His daughter Keiko, leader of the Popular Force party in Peru, who has herself been jailed for buying votes, defended her father on the sterilizations, claiming during her series of lectures in 2015 across the US at universities as disparate as Harvard and Utah Valley, that sterilizations were intended to be voluntary and that health care workers were overzealous.[29]

In each of these examples, officials rhetorically distanced themselves from the racist legacies of eugenics past. (And those weren't the only instances; the US took a keen interest in population control in Southeast Asia and the Philippines during the Vietnam War as well as in South and Central America.) Yet the official messages remained so familiar. The wrong sorts had too many children, they said. And if those with political and economic power didn't do something about it—preferably something permanent—demographic trends would upset the global status quo, and the least of these would inherit the earth. Civilization itself was at stake.

Eventually, though, at least in Europe and the US, formal eugenics programs did come to an end. Surely there are no population control programs operating in these countries anymore, are there?

PART 5

Eugenics Is Dead;
Long Live Eugenics

(1980 TO PRESENT)

CHAPTER 18

Resistance, Weak and Strong

In one of those inexplicable historical accidents that later appears to be designed, the ABC television network interrupted their Sunday night broadcast of *Judgment at Nuremberg* on March 7, 1965, to show Alabama police beating civil rights protesters crossing the Edmund Pettus Bridge in Selma. What made this interruption even more incredible is a key scene near the conclusion of *Judgment at Nuremberg*. The prosecution calls a man to the stand, a man Nazi doctors sterilized because he was feebleminded. Yet when the German defense attorney makes his argument before the American tribunal judges (the chief justice is played by Spencer Tracy), he points out that Americans had also sterilized thousands for the very same reason. *Judgment at Nuremberg* is about Nazi crimes. But the film slices through that simplistic narrative that World War II was about winning a just war against fascist villains. More than that, the juxtaposition of American cops beating hymn-singing men and women whose major crime appeared to be Marching While Black—including the future senator John Lewis—made it hard to tell where that victory in Germany twenty years earlier got us.[1] Some of the estimated 48 million viewers that night explicitly understood the connection: "I have just witnessed on television the new sequel to Adolf Hitler's brown shirts," one wrote to the *Birmingham*

News. "They were George Wallace's blue shirts. The scene in Alabama looked like scenes on old newsreels of Germany in the 1930s."[2]

According to some historians, moments like the Nuremberg Trials and Selma's Bloody Sunday permanently discredited scientific racism and eugenics.[3] At least as important, the sort of hard biological determinism underlined back in the nineteenth century by Gobineau, then championed by Sir Francis Galton, among others, finally received its comeuppance. American state judges, attorneys, and legislators repealed eugenics laws that had been on the books for decades; they were hardly in use by the 1960s anyway. Medical boards and hospitals locked down standards for treatment; no more vigilante surgeries. *One Flew Over the Cuckoo's Nest* (the 1962 novel and 1975 film) and other popular expressions of disgust at unethical uses of medical power took aim at the entire asylum system. Today, in all medical research, patients (or caregivers on the patients' behalf) must give consent. There are review boards, regulations, paperwork, and strings attached to grant money.

This, anyway, is the story we like to tell. In reality, the purported death of eugenics started far earlier. But it also took much, much longer. And some of us aren't convinced it's really dead.

The Conflicted Geneticists

While literary figures like Sinclair Lewis, for example, and legal warriors like Clarence Darrow bashed eugenics in the 1920s, scientific resistance to eugenics was never strong or persistent until the 1960s.[4]

There were, however, a few notable exceptions. In the 1920s, Herbert S. Jennings, a prominent microbiologist at

Johns Hopkins University, took the stand before the House Committee on Immigration and Naturalization, chaired by the white supremacist Albert Johnson, and disagreed with Harry H. Laughlin and those who asserted that immigration would markedly increase the proportion of criminals, epileptics, or the feebleminded in the US.[5] Jennings resigned his earlier membership in the Eugenics Society but expressed his views tepidly, and Congress ignored him.[6]

Raymond Pearl, a biologist at Johns Hopkins University, followed his mentor, Jennings, and gave a much stronger denunciation. But he paid a price for it. Pearl had been an early vocal *advocate* of eugenics, writing in the widely circulating *World's Work* magazine in 1908, "When men shall come to have as great repugnance to the multiplication of physically and mentally defective individuals as they now have toward incest, one great end of eugenics will have been gained."[7] But a few years later, his friend H. L. Mencken convinced Pearl to write an *anti*-eugenics article for *The American Mercury*. "The Biology of Superiority," Pearl called it.

In the article, Pearl chipped away at the foundations of the eugenics movement as only a turncoat insider could. Almost all eugenics literature was nonsense, insisted Pearl. He demonstrated it by conducting a survey of 588 great scholars, artists, poets, and scientists. Surely these "greats" had great parents! But Pearl found something quite *ordinary*—aggressively mediocre parents. And in many cases, quite abysmal ones—so bad that modern eugenicists would certainly have seriously considered sterilizing them. And here's another funny thing: The children of the "greats" turned out to be not so extraordinary. So, despite eugenics dogma, the likelihood of profound talent *did not* regularly pass from parent to child, as Galton insisted decades earlier after conducting a survey very similar to, though less comprehensive than, Pearl's.[8] The pathways between the genotypes (genomes on the inside) and phenotypes (what you get on the outside) are just way too complex to make predictions. So, Pearl warned, any gene-makes-trait story trumpeted by eugenicists is, at best, an oversimplification.

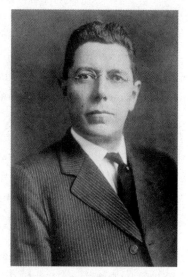

Raymond Pearl, turncoat eugenicist

For this critique, the notable geneticists and eugenics supporters Edward M. East and E. B. Wilson blacklisted Pearl.[9] He ceased to be a major voice in American biology after that point.

In the end, only anthropologists—and let's be more specific, only *cultural* anthropologists following in the footsteps of the venerable Franz Boas of Columbia University—really put their shoulders to the wheel of tearing down scientific racism and, as a byproduct, eugenics.[10] Boas's students, including Ruth Fulton Benedict, Zora Neale Hurston, Margaret Mead, Melville J. Herskovits, and M. Ashley Montagu all hacked away at the scientific support for the biological race concept that supported eugenics the way suspension cables hold up a bridge. Eventually, they were successful. At least partially. While scientific support for antisemitism precipitously declined after World War II and support for the testing of intelligence quotient (IQ) scholastic aptitude (SAT), and the psychological apparatus meant to reinforce eugenics faltered for a time, eugenic sterilizations did not disappear.[11]

The "Mississippi Appendectomy"

In 1964, less than a year before he was beaten by Alabama State Police in Selma, John Lewis wrote a newspaper editorial to raise awareness of a recently introduced piece of eugenics legislation in Mississippi. A "Genocide Bill" is what Lewis, chair of the Student Nonviolent Coordinating Committee (SNCC) in Atlanta called Mississippi House Bill 180.[12] Lewis highlighted an SNCC pamphlet, "Genocide in Mississippi," which exposed the true nature of Mississippi's intended legislation. Introduced by Representative W. B. Meek and several others early in 1964—but supported behind the scenes by the rabid segregationist Senator James O. Eastland—the bill made

it a felony for anyone to become the parent of more than one child out of wedlock. Conviction meant over a year in prison. A second "offense" tacked on three to five years. Debate was fierce, but HB 180 passed two-to-one after the legislature amended the bill to provide for a way to avoid imprisonment altogether, following the suggestion of Representative Ted

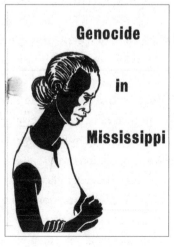

SNCC's *Genocide in Mississippi*

McCullough, a Baptist deacon and cotton merchant: The accused should undergo eugenic sterilization.

Lewis raised the alarm because of some telling quotes that Mississippi legislators let slip during the debates. Some feared that the state had a "welfare problem," and that upper-crust whites were no longer willing to "pay for it." Others admitted that HB 180 would specifically force African Americans out of the state. Representative Stone Barefield of Hattiesburg laid it bare: "When the cutting starts, [African Americans will] head for Chicago."[13] Since Black marriages were not always recognized by the state, thousands of children would become "illegitimate" at the stroke of a pen, and their parents, felons— therefore subject to imprisonment and/or sterilization. If that weren't enough, in the same 1964 session of the Mississippi legislature, Representative Fred Jones, the former superinten- dent of the Mississippi State Penitentiary, introduced HB 788, "An Act to Provide for the Sexual Sterilization of Habitual Criminals."[14] Even in the middle of the belated national awak- ening around civil rights issues, even with the recognition of Nazi atrocities, even with national media reporting on anti- Black violence and white vigilantism, even with sympathetic legislators attempting to break apart Jim Crow, sterilization measures that disproportionally affected African Americans continued to be pushed through the 1960s.

And much more happened behind physicians' closed doors, legislation or no.

When the civil rights activist Fannie Lou Hamer addressed the Women's International League of Peace and Freedom in 1964, she revealed that she had been given the "Mississippi appendectomy." In 1961, a white physician removed a "small tumor" from Hamer's uterus, suspected after two failed pregnancies. But, without Hamer's knowledge or consent while she was unconscious, the supposedly minor procedure turned into a removal of her entire uterus. She thought about suing him but decided a lawsuit against a white surgeon in Mississippi "would have been taking my hands and screwing tacks into my own casket."[15]

Still, Hamer knew her experience was not unique and that, in the case of eugenics, law often lurked along behind already existing practice. In 1965 alone, between fifty and sixty Black women at Mississippi's North Sunflower County Hospital gave birth and later learned they had been sterilized. Whether their children were thought to be "legitimate" or not had no discernable relationship to the surgeon's decision to cut.[16]

> "One of the other things that happened in . . . the North Sunflower County Hospital, I would say about six out of the ten Negro women that go to the hospital are sterilized with the tubes tied. They are getting up a law that said if a woman has an illegitimate baby and then a second one, they could draw time for six months or a five-hundred-dollar fine [HB 180]. What they didn't tell is that they are already doing these things, not only to single women but to married women."
>
> —Fannie Lou Hamer, speaking about her experience with the "Mississippi Appendectomy"[17]

Skinner v. Oklahoma Wasn't the End of Eugenics

Legal scholars have made much of *Skinner v. Oklahoma* (1942) and the opinion of Justice William O. Douglas.[18] "The power to sterilize, if exercised, may have subtle, far-reaching and devastating effects," Douglas warned during World War II. "In evil or reckless hands, it can cause races or types which are inimical to the dominant group to wither and disappear." As Justice Douglas presumably did not know, Third Reich leaders had kicked into gear their "Final Solution" at the Wannsee Conference only a few months before Douglas tolled this death knell for Oklahoma's inmate sterilization program. From 1935 to the *Skinner* decision seven years later, Oklahoma sterilized roughly sixty-five criminals per year. After *Skinner*, punitive sterilizations for inmates largely ceased—for a time.[19]

But outside the prison, *Skinner v. Oklahoma* barely registered—not at a national level or even in Oklahoma, as we'll see below.[20] However celebrated the decision in *Skinner*—and the case is historic: it would reprise its role in *Roe v. Wade* (1973)—the US Supreme Court did not rule on eugenic sterilization itself, preferring only to slice off Oklahoma's *punitive* deployment of involuntary sterilization in prisons.

CHAPTER 19

From Population Control to Poverty Control

President Johnson's Economic Opportunity Act (1964), a key feature of the War on Poverty, expanded access to voluntary birth control through Community Action Committees. After Nixon signed the Public Health Services Act in 1970, these services came to the poorest and most segregated parts of the country, such as Montgomery County, Alabama.[1] (Ironically, Nixon went on to gut much of Johnson's Great Society programs intended to help the same populations.) A series of high-profile cases demonstrated that long after the term "eugenics" and the ideas of societal degeneration had been buried, the old medical impulse to solve social problems by controlling the reproduction of the poor and undeserving continued inside the boundaries of the US. Once brought to light by the media and concerned citizen action groups in the 1970s, states and hospitals began to draw back from coerced sterilizations and to formally renounce eugenics.

> "Extreme hereditarian fervor of the early part of the century is gone, but some of this zeal and in many cases the same kind of arguments is coming to the surface again in the attacks on the recipients of public

> assistance, ADC aid, or the poor in general. One could almost say that just as our recurrent national phobia [or] hatred of the foreigner or the stranger or the group on the make in American society brings out the 'worst' in us, so, too, contempt for the weak and downtrodden has its recurring themes in American social, political, and intellectual history."
>
> —Julius Paul, early researcher into the history of eugenics (1965)[2]

Relf v. Weinberger (1973)

Soon after it received federal funds, the Montgomery Community Action Committee (MCAC) identified Lonnie and Minne Relf and their six children as candidates for aid. The MCAC helped relocate the Relfs to the new Smiley Court public housing project on the southwestern outskirts of Montgomery, Alabama, and got them registered for federally funded benefits totaling around 150 dollars per month, including regular visits from social workers and nurses. Beginning in 1971 and about every three months afterward, health care workers shuttled Katie (the oldest Relf girl, age thirteen in 1971) to a physician and family planning clinic in town. There Katie received health care checkups and an injection of Depo-Provera, a birth control serum made from the hormone progesterone (and still in regular use today). Her sisters, Mary Alice (eleven in 1971) and Minnie Lee (nine in 1971), began receiving the injection sometime later.

Upjohn Co., the manufacturer of Depo-Provera, had already received FDA approval for the drug to treat irregular uterine bleeding, endometriosis, and (strangely) certain cancers and was in the middle of a safety and efficacy study using dogs and monkeys. But no long-term human trial had been conducted. Perhaps it seemed not to be necessary: The FDA had already signaled to Upjohn that it would allow them to market Depo-Provera as a female contraceptive, which the agency confirmed in October 1973. Yet even while the FDA moved forward, physicians' anecdotes hinted that, far from being an effective treatment, the drug actually *caused* cervical cancer.[3] The cancer concern kept the FDA from fully approving Depo-Provera until 1992, but the Relf sisters had received it regularly two decades before that approval. So did hundreds of other women around the globe.

Those cancer rumors did reach the Department of Health, Education, and Welfare (HEW) and, eventually, Dr. Joseph Conklin Sr., director of the MCAC clinic in Alabama. So, in March 1974, an MCAC nurse took now sixteen-year-old Katie not for another injection of Depo-Provera but to receive a long-term IUD. Three months later, an MCAC worker returned for Katie's two younger sisters, Mary Alice (now fourteen) and Minnie Lee (now twelve)—as too many Smiley Court boys were "hanging around the girls" and it was decided these younger girls needed to continue birth control as well. But perhaps especially because Minnie Lee exhibited physical and mental disabilities, the MCAC did not want her to have children. Social workers again approached Mrs. Relf and convinced her to allow the two younger girls to be taken to Montgomery Hospital with her, where they all were "briefed on the effects of the operation," according to Conklin. Though unable to read, Mrs. Relf signed her "X" on the forms presented to her by hospital staff. A notary "quizzed" her about whether she knew what she was signing and raised no objections. An MCAC worker then took Mrs. Relf home.[4] The next morning, physicians sterilized Mary Alice and Minnie Lee by tubal ligation. After the girls recovered, MCAC workers brought them home and attempted to fetch Katie. But Katie fought back, eventually locking herself in her room, clearly frightened by what had happened to her sisters.

Within two weeks, and with the assistance of African American MCAC social workers, the Relfs contacted the Southern Poverty Law Center (SPLC), also in Montgomery. Joseph Levin Jr. (cofounder, with Morris Dees, of the SPLC) filed an attention-grabbing one-million-dollar lawsuit against the federal government, alleging that the Relf sisters had been human guinea pigs for Depo-Provera, which had still not been approved by the FDA, and that neither they nor their mother had been able to provide informed consent before the girls were sterilized. Levin upped the suit to five million dollars and added HEW Secretary Caspar Weinberger as a defendant after Levin discovered a bizarre fight inside the government regarding guidelines that would have better regulated the sterilization operations on the girls, and maybe even prevented them. Rather than distributing twenty-five thousand copies of the new guidelines on the use of medical treatments on the mentally handicapped, which were in fact written and approved in 1972, the HEW stashed them in a warehouse, allowing the sterilizations to continue unregulated.[5]

Growing numbers of news stories uncovered involuntary "appendectomies" performed on African American women in Los Angeles (1968), Boston (1972), and South Carolina (1972), as well as the steady trickle of stories out of Virginia and North Carolina through the 1960s and early '70s.[6] And, given the recent revelations around the Tuskegee syphilis trials, continued rumors of atrocities in Southeast Asia, and the steady drumbeat surrounding the Watergate scandal—the example of government malfeasance in Montgomery resonated with a national press already suspicious of the Nixon administration.[7] Senator Ted Kennedy (D-Massachusetts) caught wind of the case and invited the Relfs to testify before a Senate subcommittee. Kennedy hoped the testimony would jump-start his bill for a law preventing medical experimentation on unwitting individuals—though even in Kennedy's hearing, no one explicitly mentioned eugenics or the sterilization of the unfit.[8] Politically, it worked. Kennedy's National Research Act was signed into law in 1974, creating a National Commission for the Protection of Human Subjects of Biomedical and Behavioral Research.[9] That agency's "Belmont Report" outlining ethics in biomedicine followed soon after. *Relf v. Weinberger* (1973) joined *Skinner v. Oklahoma* (1942), *Loving v. Virginia* (1967), and other landmark cases against the old practice of the powerful controlling the reproduction of the marginalized.

Madrigal v. Quilligan (1975)

Consuelo Hermosillo agreed under duress to be sterilized by tubal ligation at the Los Angeles County USC Medical Center (LAC-USC) at nearly the same moment medical authorities in Alabama did the same thing to the Relf sisters. While Hermosillo was in labor, a nurse told her she could not have the C-section she needed to save her baby's life unless she also submitted to sterilization afterward. Hermosillo signed, much like Mrs. Relf did thousands of miles to the east. As a whistleblower soon revealed, such ultimatums to Hispanic women giving birth had become a trend at that hospital—which also happened to be the exterior shot for the popular soap opera *General Hospital*. In fact, over the 1960s and into the '70s, California medical workers routinely coerced working-class Mexican American women into postpartum tubal ligations hours or even minutes after undergoing cesarean deliveries.[10] "The doctor would hold a syringe in front of the mother who was in labor and ask her if she wanted a painkiller," a concerned physician later reported. "While the woman was in the throes of a contraction the doctor would say, 'Do you want the painkiller? Then sign the papers.'"[11] Another resident at LAC-USC, Dr. Bernard Rosenfeld, began to feel distressed by the hundreds of coerced sterilizations going on there. While making copies of medical records, he noted a 400 percent increase in tubal ligations and hysterectomies from 1968 through the early '70s, often performed on Mexican American women.[12] After publishing these findings in a 1973 report, Rosenfeld passed the records to Antonia Hernández at the nearby Los Angeles Center for Law & Justice.[13] More of these sorts of stories reverberated through the Mexican American community on the east side of LA, and Hernández convinced Hermosillo and eight other women to join Dolores Madrigal (the "Madrigal Ten," as they were called) in a class action lawsuit against LAC-USC chief residents and others, even naming, as in *Relf*, HEW Secretary Weinberger. *Madrigal v. Quilligan* (1975) became another landmark case contributing to the 1970s death of American eugenics.[14]

But physicians' groups pushed back. Judge Jesse Curtis, the Nixon appointee who came in from his yacht each day to preside over the trial, decided that *Madrigal et al.* were

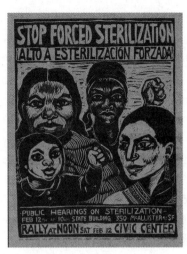

Madrigal v. Quilligan case

victims of their own ignorance. The physicians followed their training and experience, pursuing the best for their patients. More disturbingly, Curtis seemed to suggest that sterilization to address the "overpopulation problem" was perfectly legitimate, provided that physicians didn't "overpower" their patients.[15] Despite the plaintiffs' loss in court, *Madrigal v. Quilligan* did inspire lasting change. California adopted bilingual sterilization consent forms and a seventy-two-hour waiting period between consent and surgery. Perhaps most important, the California Department of Health approved a signed consent statement with an acknowledgment that welfare benefits would not be denied if a patient refused to consent.[16]

Indian Health Care Improvement Act (1976)

Norma Jean Serena of Armstrong County, Pennsylvania, had five children. The delivery of her fifth, Shawn, in 1970 turned out to be more difficult than the previous four. As she lay in her hospital bed the next day, still exhausted and hazy from medication, nurses asked her to sign some papers. Sterilization papers. For her best interest, and given that future pregnancies "might result in the birth of retarded or deformed children," the Pittsburgh hospital physicians had sterilized Serena just after Shawn's birth.[17] Let me underscore that point: Consent *followed* the surgery. Children's Services soon removed Shawn from Serena's care. In 1973, with the aid of the Three Rivers American Indian Center, Serena filed suit and won back custody. The sterilizations, however, were another matter.

"I'm sure the facts of her case are not uncommon," Serena's attorney, Richard Levine, said with a sigh. Norma Jean Serena was Creek-Shawnee from Oklahoma, originally. By the mid-1970s, the Association of American Indian Affairs sounded the alarm that one in seven Native women had been sterilized, often without any consent or even recognition that the surgery happened.[18] It may not have been intentional bigotry, but it seemed to observers that the US was punishing Native American women for their own poverty and cultural marginalization.

From 1973 to 1975, members of the Public Citizen's Health Research Group (PCHRG) surveyed hospitals in Boston, Baltimore, and Southern California to determine physicians' attitudes toward sterilization. The PCHRG discovered that, with the introduction of LBJ's War on Poverty programs, white surgeons believed they were unfairly shouldering a larger tax burden to pay for Medicaid and other forms of welfare for low-income non-whites. They recognized that they had a duty to care not only for their patients' immediate health needs but also for society's longer-term well-being. And if that happened to coincide with lowering their own taxes, so much the better. This led to behaviors that the PCHRG called "the hard sell" of sterilization procedures to non-white women. Under the guise of "voluntary" and "consensual" sterilization procedures, medical interns and residents at these hospitals systematically violated fundamental patient rights.[19] In one Baltimore hospital, for instance, a dozen African American women were handed multipage sterilization consent forms just minutes before receiving C-section deliveries. Residents at a California hospital approached women at the same moment of duress, "asking the women whether they wanted to go through this pain again."[20] By the 1970s, the number of Black women who had been sterilized in Boston, Baltimore, and Los Angeles tripled that of white women, the PCHRG uncovered. Some of these women told the PCHRG that health care workers would hold their newly delivered babies threateningly and demand that the mother sign sterilization paperwork before being handed her child.[21]

Once again, physicians didn't see these practices as manipulative or discriminatory at all. By conducting tubal ligations, salpingectomies, and hysterectomies, these doctors assumed that they were meeting their professional duties, helping minority women by reducing mouths to feed, and helping cut the need for Medicaid, which would have the happy effect of lessening physicians' own personal taxes. Many also directly increased their own personal income by performing these surgeries on minority women: Surgeries earned more than prescribing a contraceptive pill that the physician didn't believe poor non-white patients would faithfully take (echoes of Puerto Rico).[22] Many younger surgeons owned up to the fact that they sterilized to gain valuable experience in gynecological surgery. It didn't bother them that they were operating on the federal government's dime. As one physician noted, "Enthusiasm for performing sterilization by elective vaginal hysterectomy and cesarean hysterectomy in the name of residency training is commonplace in some university hospitals."[23]

But among Native American mothers, historically some of the most vulnerable people in the US, few could deny that a kind of eugenics persisted. "The destruction of Native Peoples, as peoples, is part of a much larger program of the United States," said John Mohawk, University of Buffalo professor and activist for the cultural survival of indigenous peoples, and he did not just mean this in reference to the seventeenth-century colonization stories or the nineteenth-century "Indian Wars."[24] He meant it was still happening, right then in the 1970s. The US government and white physicians across the country were still attempting to eliminate Native Americans, now by sterilizing their women and confiscating their children.

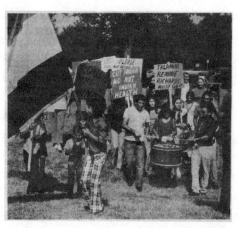

Indigenous demonstrators protest involuntary sterilization procedures at an IHS facility in Claremore, Oklahoma.

In the early 1970s, Dr. Connie Redbird Pinkerman-Uri, a California anesthesiologist and Indian Health Service (IHS) advocate, heard rumors of coerced hysterectomies at a Claremore, Oklahoma, hospital—one of a handful that served women from a dozen Native American tribes in northeast Oklahoma, thirty miles outside Tulsa.[25] Over a series of interviews in August 1974, she learned that "for every four Indian babies born, one woman was sterilized."[26] Doctors sterilized over one hundred Native American women there in 1973 alone.[27] It felt like continued displacement and threatened destruction of Native Americans by whites.[28] Dr. Pinkerman-Uri didn't see this larger pattern of involuntary and coerced sterilizations, however, until she was able to examine the surgical records book. When she first requested the book, it had "gone missing." Only when she sought help in Washington did the surgical records reappear—in the possession of Dr. William Gideon, the hospital's chief of staff.[29]

Continued pressure by Dr. Pinkerman-Uri and others got the attention of Senator James Abourezk (D-South Dakota), the chair of the Senate Subcommittee on Indian affairs, and of the General Accounting Office (GAO). In 1976, the GAO reported that in just the previous three years physicians in the Oklahoma City, Phoenix, Albuquerque, and Aberdeen IHS regions carried out an astonishing 3,406 sterilizations of Native American women—3,001 of whom were of childbearing age.[30] Physicians at facilities under contract to IHS performed 1,024 of these (or around 30 percent). Almost 150 Native American men also received sterilization operations, and by all accounts, this was an undercount. In a few cases, HEW regulations put in place after *Relf v. Weinberger* (1973) also seemed not to be followed, though it was possible physicians didn't know them.[31] Even the post-*Relf* patient consent form comprised four pages of technical language. Dr. Pinkerman-Uri believed the information would be difficult to grasp by the average woman about to be sterilized. Far too many women reported that the forms, if presented at all, were shoved in their faces in moments of duress. If that was considered consent, it certainly couldn't have been thoughtfully given.[32]

The combination of calls for justice by Dr. Pinkerman-Uri and the PCHRG, plus the 1976 GAO report, did spur the federal government to act. In 1976, Congress passed the Indian Health Care Improvement Act (IHCIA). Title V of IHCIA organized specific Urban Indian Organizations (UIOs) to be responsible for providing culturally appropriate health care facilities in cities outside any reservation. The IHS and its UIOs continue to provide medical, dental, and vision care, alcohol and drug abuse prevention, AIDS and STD education and prevention, mental health services, nutrition education and counseling services, pharmacy services, and home health care to indigenous populations today.[33] After funding for the IHCIA stumbled in Republican-led Congresses for over a decade, Democrats under President Barack Obama permanently reauthorized funding it as part of the Affordable Care Act ("Obamacare") in 2010.[34]

National Struggles Through the 1970s

Still, the national tug-of-war over sterilizations lasted through the 1970s. Civil rights organizations, such as the New York–based Committee to End Sterilization Abuse (CESA), pushed hard to force a national statute on age limitations, consent documents, multilingual explanatory paperwork, and waiting periods. CESA and other groups repeatedly called to account governments, hospitals, and state health departments when providers failed to follow the provisions that emerged out of the court cases.[35] At the same time, the work of historians such as Donald Pickens, Kenneth M. Ludmerer, Mark Adams, and Garland Allen pried open the closet of the American medical community to expose those old eugenics skeletons.[36] Finally, powerful people paid attention.

While there was sporadic repeal of state eugenics legislation through the middle of the century, public pressure for more started in earnest in the wake of the civil rights cases in the 1970s. Legislatures in both Virginia, where the law that led to *Buck v. Bell* originated, and Indiana, the state that passed the first American sterilization law in 1907, repealed their eugenics laws in 1974. The California State Legislature unanimously repealed its law—which had legalized over twenty thousand nonconsensual procedures since 1909—in 1979. Eugenics laws crumbled through the next two decades in North and South Carolina, Kansas, Nebraska, North and South Dakota, New Jersey, and Oregon, and even in West Virginia, which dithered until 2013.[37] Others, including Connecticut, Missouri, Maine, Alabama, Delaware, and Maryland, rewrote statutes to make sterilization of the disabled much more difficult. And in November 1978, HEW changed its own policies after years of lawsuits. Federal funds, such as Medicare or the social services programs administered by Nixon-era Public Health Services, could no longer be used to sterilize persons under twenty-one years of age, mentally incompetent persons, or institutionalized persons no matter what age. Now, just as CESA had worked for, patients need to sign a special consent form, written in the patient's primary language, with a thirty-day wait before any sterilization procedure.[38] Pressure groups forced states like North Carolina and Virginia to issue formal apologies, and even to offer compensation for those involuntarily sterilized.

At long last, more than a generation after Nazi eugenics was exposed in Europe, a half century after "three generations of imbeciles are enough," and eight decades after Harry Sharp's knife cut into "Clawson," the inmate in at the Jeffersonville Asylum in Indiana, eugenics was dead.

At least, that's the story we tell ourselves.

Whose Choice?

By March 1981, just a few weeks into the Reagan administration, Texas was already feeling drastic cuts to services for the poor. Lyndon Johnson's home state of Texas rejected his Great Society by cutting spending on its poorest by over 20 percent, pushing it below levels that had been considered necessary throughout the previous decade.[39] A tax-cut fan, Houston's state senator Walter H. Mengden Jr. sensed an opportunity. He sent an extensive questionnaire to his constituents, asking about "euthanasia for the elderly and terminally ill," "painlessly killing permanently ill mental patients in state institutions," and, in an infamous question number 40, whether women on welfare with two children should be *automatically* sterilized.[40] When constituents, newspapers, and other legislators balked at his questions, Mengden defended himself, saying he was attempting to gather Texans' opinions regarding "life that some people might regard as an undesirable burden to society."[41] He never picked up on the Nazi connotation. Instead, Mengden defiantly maintained that "the sterilization of welfare moms question" couldn't have been controversial, since many powerful Texans that he knew personally held that view.

It's true that mentally and physically impaired individuals ceased being the primary target of eugenic surgeries in the last quarter of the twentieth century. Yet those with social status still held convictions about controlling the reproduction of the marginalized—because such control benefited society, they said. When asked in a national poll what should be done with unwed mothers on welfare who had children, 50 percent of Americans surveyed by Gallup said they should lose welfare benefits. The second most frequent answer—totaling one in five respondents—was "sterilize the women."[42]

> "Sometimes unwed mothers on relief continue to have illegitimate children and get relief money for each new child born. What do you think should be done in the case of these women? How about the children?"
>
> The suggestions offered most frequently by about half of the persons interviewed in this survey was to "stop giving them relief money."
> Next most often mentioned, by roughly one person in five, was "sterilize the women."

Gallup poll advocating sterilization of welfare mothers
(*The Washington Post*, January 1965)

CHAPTER 20

Sterilizing Criminals Again

"A re Some Criminals Born That Way?" asked Dr. Mary Telfer, a biochemist, conducting research at the Elwyn Institute in Pennsylvania (formerly the Pennsylvania Training School for Feeble-Minded Children, site of over 250 eugenic sterilizations). She had recently identified a curious trait in one of her Black patients. As a follow-up, she and three colleagues tested 129 institutionalized criminals. Almost 10 percent possessed the same trait as her original patient: a feeblemindedness connected to criminality.[1] You could see the physiological stigmata on their faces, pockmarked with acne scars, and their over-long limbs. She maintained they were the classic criminal type: sexually motivated, physically overpowering, and mentally unstable—degenerates. So, *yes*, said Telfer, natural born criminals *are* out there.

But this wasn't some study from the nineteenth century criminal anthropology era of Lombroso; Telfer conducted this study in the 1960s. From her position at the Elwyn Institute, she found that these tall criminals possessed a discrete criminal *essence*, an extra Y-chromosome.[2] This finding matched up with an earlier study published in the venerable journal *Nature* that found nine men in a high-security mental institution in Scotland with "dangerous, violent or criminal propensities," who all possessed the same extra Y-chromosome abnormality.[3]

Criminal anthropology faded, yes. But the notion of the born criminal carrying an inherited propensity to crime, an idea that haunted physicians and prison wardens in the late nineteenth century and seeding American eugenics in the twentieth, never quite disappeared. It is true that *Skinner v. Oklahoma* (1942) made punitive sterilization illegal in Oklahoma. It's also true that present-day cases of punitive sterilization are fewer in number than they were in the mid-twentieth century. Nevertheless, punitive surgical solutions still exist for criminals, just as they did in the days of Harry Sharp in Indiana.

Dr. Tefler's "XYY syndrome" exploded in popularity among psychologists and geneticists all through the late 1960s and early '70s, with many studies of already incarcerated patients showing that some percentage had that extra Y-chromosome. Richard Speck, the serial killer who murdered eight student nurses in Chicago in 1966, was said to be a classic case of XYY syndrome (he wasn't).[4] *Time, Newsweek*, and *The New York Times*, among many other outlets, all reported breathlessly on the syndrome, including stories of attorneys invoking XYY syndrome to defend their clients.[5] Just as Dr. Jekyll/Mr. Hyde and Dracula once popularized the hereditary criminal, crime dramas like *Law & Order* and *CSI: Miami* stoked the same fears in the late twentieth century.[6] Perhaps most memorably, in *Alien 3* (1992) Sigourney Weaver's character, Ellen Ripley, crash-lands in an outer space penal colony filled with XYY criminals too violent to incarcerate elsewhere.[7]

After being repeatedly debunked, XYY crime worries were soon replaced by the equally dubious notion of "superpredators"—deviant youths devoid of a moral conscious. In the

1990s, John J. DiIulio Jr., a political scientist then at Princeton (and now at the University of Pennsylvania) and James Alan Fox, a professor of criminology at Northeastern University, predicted "a blood bath of violence" by superpredators.[8] So convincing were their dire warnings that First Lady Hillary Rodham Clinton repeated them on-air in support of the 1994 crime bill.[9] Studies later debunked the idea of "superpredators," however.

Yet so thirsty were elites for hereditary crime to be true, that twenty-first-century criminologists, politicians, and the public latched on to another criminal essence. This one was a genetic mutation of an enzyme called monoamine oxidase A (MAOA). MAOA regulates the function of neurotransmitters. And men who possessed an MAOA mutation expressed suspiciously similar behavioral patterns to that of the mythological XYY syndrome men: aggressive, even violent, and somewhat mentally impaired.[10] Scientists published dozens and dozens of peer-reviewed papers on the subject over the rest of the decade. Biological anthropologists offhandedly dubbed the MAOA mutation the "warrior gene," speculating that, since it appeared in some ape lineages and in a high percentage of Māori men in New Zealand, it must convey some sort of long-term selective advantage for aggression.[11] As with "superpredator" and the "XYY supermale," the news and entertainment media gobbled up "warrior genes"—even long after other studies had discredited this concept.[12]

In the US, aside from serial killers, depictions of XYY men were almost always tall, incarcerated Black men. The media portrayed superpredators as Black youth in Chicago. Warrior genes were carried by non-white populations as well. As a result, authorities expanded police forces, lengthened sentences, and sent more—and younger—racial minorities to prison.[13] In 1970, before the XYY criminal image took hold in the American imagination, approximately 96 out of every 100,000 Americans were in a US state or federal prison. By the beginning of the Great Recession in 2008, that number jumped to 506 per 100,000—a number and a pace of locking people up never before seen in world history. To some legal scholars, the impacts of biologizing crime, along with harsh confinement, closely mimics eugenics—effectively removing these individuals from the gene pool.[14]

Castration, albeit largely pharmaceutical and potentially reversible, appeared again as a viable punishment at the same time as, and in direct response to, fears of biologically determined criminals. In the mid-70s, Johns Hopkins University researchers injected thirteen young Black men deemed aggressive, "antisocial, and/or sex-offending" with Depo-Provera, the same controversial drug used on the Relf sisters in Alabama.[15] The treatment showed only mild effectiveness for inhibiting their sexual impulses, and the treatment was halted, perhaps because one of the subjects committed suicide.[16] Nevertheless, legislatures still passed statutes allowing for chemical castration using the drug.

At first, courts resisted the use of drugs for chemical castration. However, the US Supreme Court in *Washington v. Harper* (1990) upheld forcible administration of antipsychotic medication to prison inmates, and states have increasingly returned to the promise of intervening in the reproductive capabilities of criminals. In 1996, California legalized inmate sterilization, and, as news of deviants continued to agitate the public, legislatures and governors in Texas, Hawaii, Idaho, New Mexico, Washington, Wisconsin, Florida, Mississippi,

Tennessee, Arizona, Colorado, and Michigan immediately considered following California's lead.[17]

Legal challenges followed. Attorneys raised "no cruel and unusual punishment," of course.[18] Critics also immediately focused on chemical castration's unequal effect on men and women, thereby violating the Equal Protection Clause.[19] And then there were typical issues about the right to privacy and bodily integrity brought up all the way back in *Skinner v. Oklahoma* (1942).[20] Moreover, the psychiatric community admitted they did not understand "sexual offenses or sexual offenders" well enough to know how such a treatment might work toward deterrence.[21] Still, the laws went forward. As the newly developed Center for Sex Offender Management (CSOM), led by the Center for Effective Public Policy (CEPP) and supported by the US Department of Justice, Office of Justice Programs, maintained, sex crimes were on the rise and prisons were overcrowded with sexual predators.[22] Beyond that, CSOM insisted that more than one in three child molesters would repeat their crimes; they put the recidivism rate for rapists even higher at an astounding 46.2 percent nationally.[23] In the first decade of the twenty-first century, America appeared to be in the throes of a sex crime epidemic, and something drastic needed to be done.

In 2013, the Center for Investigative Reporting revealed that doctors had surgically sterilized almost 150 incarcerated women at two California facilities between 2006 and 2010 either without their knowledge or under coercion.[24] Anecdotal evidence from former inmates and guards suggested that, in truth, far more had been involuntarily sterilized. Many reported being pressured to consent by James Heinrich, an obstetrician/gynecologist at Valley State Prison in Chowchilla. Heinrich made his views clear, unintention-ally parroting an old eugenics line: "Over a ten-year period, [the cost of the surgeries] isn't a huge amount of money com-pared to what you save in welfare paying for these unwanted children—as they procreated more."[25] When informed by the California Prison Health Care Receivership Review Commit-tee in 2010 that California would not pay for these sorts of "not medically necessary" surgeries, health care professionals reacted with anger. The doctors did not believe they needed permission to sterilize inmates. "Everybody was operating on the fact that this was a perfectly reasonable thing to do," the Review Committee director said.[26] Still, distressed by how much this situation resembled eugenic sterilizations of days gone by, California banned such procedures on inmates in State Bill 1135 in 2014.[27]

Outside California, more American states have retained or adopted chemical castration laws in recent years. And judges have gone out on their own to make criminal steri-lization a sentencing option. In 2017, a judge in White County, Tennessee, offered to reduce sentences by thirty days if men agreed to a vasectomy or women to a contra-ception implant.[28] (The judge rescinded the order shortly thereafter, once national media caught word of it.)[29] A year later, US District Judge Stephen Friot reduced the sentence of an Oklahoma woman with a list of small crimes, a history of habitual drug use, and seven children. "Ms. Creel may, if (and only if) she chooses to do so, present medical evi-dence to the court establishing that she has been rendered incapable of procreation," Judge Friot proclaimed before sentencing. And when the prosecution objected that steri-lization had nothing to do with her criminal history, Friot retorted that "the Supreme Court has yet to recognize a constitutional right to bring crack or methamphetamine addicted babies into this world."[30] Similar cases occurred in West Virginia, Virginia, and Tennessee in the 2010s.[31] Louisiana passed a new chemical castration bill in 2008; evidence suggests it was an intentionally punitive law without much thought toward therapy or even a reduction in the prison population.[32] And this was in the state with the highest incarceration rate per capita in the world.[33] Alabama belatedly followed Louisiana and other Republican strongholds, introducing its chemical castration law (AL HB379) in 2019, which would force parolees to pay for regular Depo-Provera injections until Republican-dominated courts—not physicians or psychiatrists—allowed them to stop.[34]

Some of these laws remain in active use. In 2021, Louisiana's Third Circuit Court of Appeals heard a challenge to its chemical castration statutes. Lance Barton, who had been convicted in 2015 of five counts of molestation of a juvenile under the age of five, was convicted for a second time for juvenile molestation. So, along with a fifty-year prison sentence without parole, District Judge K. D. Earles sentenced Barton to a lifetime of chemical castration treatments. After reviewing Barton's 2020 appeal, the appellate court found this not to be an excessive sentence.[35]

This decision revealed a small but persistent trend. As of 2023, Alabama, Florida, Iowa, Louisiana, Montana, Texas, Wisconsin, and the territory of Guam still had provisions allowing for the offer of, if not the demand for, hormone injections to sex offenders as conditions of parole or to reduce sentences. West Virginia is weighing a bill to allow those convicted of drug offenses to voluntarily sterilize themselves to receive a reduced sentence.[36] Russia, South Korea, Peru, Thailand, Moldova, Poland, and Indonesia have similar statutes.

Admittedly, to show that there are isolated, and sometimes not-so-isolated, moments of sterilization surgeries or Depo-Provera injections is not to show that full-blown eugenics is on our doorstep again. In the twenty-first century, surely, we know better, right?

CHAPTER 21

Newgenics?

As typically encapsulated, twentieth-century eugenics comprised an assault on the mentally disabled. And much of the expressed fear about twenty-first century "newgenics" follows from that: eliminate physically or mentally disabled embryos or enhance the genomes of the powerful few, thereby creating greater biological disparities to cement the already existing socioeconomic ones. This rebranding has been termed "velvet eugenics" because it allows for consumer choice rather than governmental coercion.

But it's not the whole story. The velvet eugenics story, as compelling as it is, merely frets about the stuff of science future in order to overlook what is happening right in front of our eyes. Given the widely reported, deep-seated skepticism of the broader public toward genetic engineering, velvet eugenics is likely a distraction.[1] Sci-fi horror lite. There is something much nearer at hand, more quotidian going on.[2]

Reports of Eugenics in 2020

"When I met all these women who had had surgeries, I thought this was like an experimental concentration camp," reported Dawn Wooten, a licensed practical nurse at the Irwin County Detention Center (ICDC) in Ocilla, Georgia, who filed a whistleblower complaint against her facility.[3] ICDC was a for-profit prison operated by LaSalle Corrections that housed hundreds of immigrant women from states thousands of miles to the west. Wooten reported inhumane conditions throughout.[4] But the part of her testimony that yanked media attention away from the other national catastrophes in 2020 was the section that detailed involuntary sterilizations conducted on these defenseless immigrant women: "It was like they're experimenting with our bodies," reported one incredulous detainee.[5] The detained women gave their physician an ominous nickname: "the uterus collector."[6]

Nurse Wooton might not have known the precise way her observations fit into the multicentury-long story of eugenics when she contacted Project South's attorneys in the summer of 2020. But she knew intuitively that something bad was occurring, something connected to a dark history. The subsequent investigation by Project South, an advocacy institute for the elimination of poverty and genocide, together with Georgia Detention Watch, the Georgia Latino Alliance for Human Rights, and the South Georgia Immigrant Support Network, revealed something simultaneously disturbing *and* completely typical—something consistent with the long international story of eugenics.[7] According to the sworn testimonies of over forty women from twenty-five different countries, including Bolivia, Cuba, Guatemala, Honduras, India, Russia, Senegal, and Somalia, the contract physician at this Immigration and Customs Enforcement (ICE) facility conducted numerous nonconsensual medical procedures on their reproductive systems. Not much had changed since the "death" of eugenics, it appeared. The physician allegedly even administered Depo-Provera without consent or explanation. And, according to the report, when the women spoke out, ICE authorities placed them in solitary confinement. The women reported physical intimidation and unprovoked assaults. Many also faced deportation.[8] ICE sent others to the Stewart Detention Center in Lumpkin, Georgia, a facility already under fire for being one of the least safe facilities in the country.[9]

In May 2021, the new Biden administration broke the contract with LaSalle Corrections, which owned ICDC. A follow-up report by the Office of Inspector General (OIG) at the US Department of Homeland Security's (DHS) in January 2022 noted that the ICDC indeed followed most stated health guidelines during COVID. But they also admitted that their own investigation was somewhat hamstrung. After the federal government ended its contract with LaSalle Corrections, ICDC and ICE transferred many of the individuals who would have been part of a broader investigation—including all of the women detainees. DHS's OIG could not follow up on "specific allegations about detainees referred for gynecological procedures" even though this was the most troubling part of the original complaint, and the part that most resembled the eugenics of the past.[10] Unfortunately, we still don't fully know what happened.

Meanwhile, people inside and outside the facility were working as hard as they could to obtain justice for the detainees. A short 2021 documentary, *The Facility*, by the journalist Seth Freed Wessler, detailed the egregious conditions at ICDC, and for those in ICE detention more generally in 2020, through the eyes of inmates.[11] But still, it took the specter of eugenics to really get the national media's attention. And only through that pressure did ICE and LaSalle Corrections take action. On November 10, 2020, just after Americans voted Trump out of office, ICE released a few individuals who had been interviewed by attorneys and by Wessler, unannounced and with no explanation. As Andrea, one of the detained women interviewed for *The Facility*, interpreted the rapid move, "Something catastrophic had to happen for people to notice us."

No Designer Babies, Just Powerless Immigrant Women

For decades now, we've been warned that newgenics is right around the corner. "Designer babies," "playing God," and altering the potential of our descendants by fiddling with our genomes using biotechnologies that have not yet been developed—these are the contentious futures predicted in novels and science fiction films, but also fretted over even by the designers of new biotech tools. Indeed, one day we might get cloned children with pristine genomes scrubbed of known hereditary illnesses. We might be able to choose greater intelligence or strength or height—or a physique formerly possible only in comic books. Maybe. Our ethics should indeed have a stake in how these biotechnologies get deployed when they appear.

The threat of eugenics *as actually experienced in history*, though, has never been about superchildren or curing diseases. In the 1870s, the Oneida Bible Commune attempted to create a more humane family with better-bred children, and actually saw some success, according to their standards. And when we discuss the eugenics movement between the World Wars, we sometimes cite "Better Baby" and "Fitter Family" contests—these, indeed, are what Sinclair Lewis mocked in his novel *Arrowsmith*. But these methods of *improvement* never stuck for long.

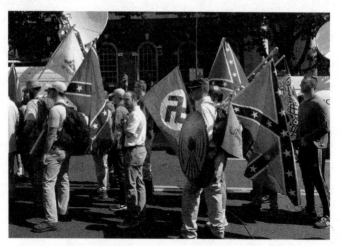

Fear of White Replacement rebounds in 2010s

Eugenics has more frequently followed Gobineau, Grant, Davenport, Laughlin, and Stoddard. Fearing degeneration, European and American eugenicists have, more often than not, walked the path of disciplining and punishing the weak and the marginalized, scorning purported love-thy-neighbor principles to do so. And American physicians continued to conduct these eugenic surgeries even *after* the menace of Nazi eugenics became well known.[12]

We are, once again, in an era of rising paranoia over white "replacement" by the "brown menace."[13] When the cutting starts again, it will not be velvet smooth. It will be on bodies of non-whites in some out-of-the-way place, some detention facility outside the purview of the federal government, maybe near the Mexican border, allowing individuals to skirt the guardrails set up in the 1970s to prevent eugenics. It may even emerge in the guise of reducing the environmental impact of humans on the planet.

Sadly, although no one can predict the future, I'm confident eugenics will reappear. Because if you find yourself in great need, and if you represent something that the white, powerful, and wealthy do not want, for you America seems always poised in a defensive crouch, always knife in hand, always right on the edge of cutting.

Notes

All sources translated by the author, unless otherwise noted.

Preface

1. Nancy Ordover, *American Eugenics: Race, Queer Anatomy, and the Science of Nationalism* (Minneapolis: University of Minnesota Press, 2003).

1. Managing Fate

1. Theognis, in D. E. Gerber (ed. and trans.), *Greek Elegiac Poetry* (Cambridge: Harvard University Press, 1999).

2. Charles Darwin, *The Descent of Man*, 2nd edition (London: John Murray, 1874).

3. M. F. Ashley Montagu, "Theognis, Darwin, and Social Selection," *Isis* 37, no. 1/2 (1947): 24–26.

4. Friedrich Nietzsche, *De Theognide Megarensi* ("On Theognis of Megara"), trans. R. M. Kerr (The Nietzsche Channel, 2015).

5. Plato, *Republic*, 5.459a–c, in *Plato in Twelve Volumes*, vol. 5, trans. Paul Shorey (Cambridge: Harvard University Press, 1969).

6. Ibid.

7. Seneca, "On Anger," Book 1, 15.2, in *Anger, Mercy, Revenge*, trans. Robert A. Kaster and Martha C. Nussbaum (Chicago: University of Chicago Press, 2010).

8. Hilda Herrick Noyes and George Wallingford Noyes, "The Oneida Community Experiment in Stirpiculture," in *Scientific Papers of the Second International Congress of Eugenics Held at the American Museum of Natural History, New York, September 22–28, 1921* (Baltimore: Williams & Wilkins Co., 1923).

9. Victoria Woodhull, "Stirpiculture; or, the Scientific Propagation of the Human Race," in Cari M. Carpenter (ed.), *Selected Writings of Victoria Woodhull: Suffrage, Free Love, and Eugenics* (Lincoln: University of Nebraska Press, 2010).

2. Degenerates

1. J. Arthur de Gobineau, *The Inequality of Human Races*, trans. Adrian Collins (London: William Heinemann, 1915).

2. Arthur Herman, *The Idea of Decline in Western History* (New York: Free Press, 1997).

3. Gerald Spring, *The Vitalism of Count de Gobineau* (New York: Institute of French Studies Press, 1932).

4. J. Arthur de Gobineau, *The Inequality of Human Races*, op. cit.

5. Nicole Hahn Rafter, "White Trash: Eugenics as Social Ideology," *Society* 26, no. 1 (November 1988): 43–49.

6. Frédéric Carbonel, "L'asile Pour Aliénés de Rouen," *Histoire & Mesure* 20, no. 1/2 (October 2005).

7. Bénédict Augustin Morel, *Mélanges d'Anthropologie Pathologique et de Médecine Mentale* (Rouen: Imprimerie de Alfred Péron, 1859).

8. Bénédict Augustin Morel, *Traité des dégénérescences physiques, intellectuelles, et morales de l'espèce humaine: et des causes qui produisent ces variétés maladives* (Paris: J.B. Baillière, 1857).

9. T. M. Porter, "Statistical and social facts from Quetelet to Durkheim," *Sociological Perspectives* 38, no. 1 (1995): 15–26.

10. Lambert Adolphe Jacques Quêtelet, *Du système social et des lois qui le régissent* (Paris: Guillamine et Cie Libraire, 1848).

11. Lambert Adolphe Jacques Quêtelet, *Sur l'homme et le développement de ses facultés, ou essai de physique sociale* (Paris: Bachelier Imprimeur-Libraire, 1835).

12. Ibid.

13. Ibid.

14. Ibid.

15. B. A. Morel, *Traité des maladies mentales* (Paris: Masson, 1860).

16. François Deherly, "Bénédict-Auguste Morel, théoricien de la dégénérescence," Le Blog Gallica, January 17, 2023, gallica.bnf.fr/blog/17012023/benedict-auguste-morel-theoricien-de-la-degenerescence.

17. Hippolyte Taine, *Les Origines de la France Contemporaine; La Révolution: II—La Conquête Jacobine* (Paris: Hachette et Cie, 1881).

18. Guillaume Ferrero, "Somme-nous Malades?," *La Revue des revues* (September 1893): 41.

3. Natural-Born Criminals

1. Pierre-Louis Moreau Maupertuis, *The Earthly Venus*, trans. Simone Brangier Boas (New York: Johnson Reprint Corp., 1966).

2. "Edward Fowler, Cotton Pioneer, Dies in Pasadena," *Pasadena Independent*, February 4, 1959, findagrave.com/memorial/163401062/edward-mumford-fowler.

3. L. N. Fowler, "The Responsibility of Criminals," *Phrenological Journal & Life Illustrated* 61, no. 3 (September 1875): 184–85.

4. E. P. Fowler, "Are the Brains of Criminals Anatomical Perversions?," *Medico-Chirurgical Quarterly* 1 (October 1880): 1–32.

5. Moritz Benedikt, *Anatomical Studies upon Brains of Criminals: A Contribution to Anthropology, Medicine, Jurisprudence, and Psychology*, trans. E. P. Fowler (New York: W. Wood, 1881).

6. Ibid.

7. "Forty Fifth Annual Report of the Inspectors of the State Penitentiary for the Eastern District of Pennsylvania for the Year 1875," Board of Inspectors of the Eastern State Penitentiary, 1875.

8. "Forty Ninth Annual Report of the Inspectors of the State Penitentiary for the Eastern District of Pennsylvania for the Year 1879," Board of Inspectors of the Eastern State Penitentiary, 1879.

9. H. G. Hayes and C. J. Hayes, *A Complete History of the Life and Trial of Charles Julius Guiteau, Assassin of President Garfield* (Philadelphia: Hubbard Bros., 1882).

10. J. G. Kiernan, "Review of *Transactions of the Pennsylvania State Medical Society*, vol. 14 (1883)," *Journal of Nervous and Mental Disease* 11, no. 2 (1884): 272–74.

11. J. J. Elwell et al., "The Moral Responsibility of the Insane," *North American Review* 134 (January 1882): 1–39.

12. Nicole Rafter et al., *The Criminal Brain: Understanding Biological Theories of Crime*, 2nd ed. (New York: NYU Press, 2016): 73.

13. Cesare Lombroso, *L'uomo bianco e l'uomo di colore, letture sull'origine e le varietà delle razze umane* (Padova, Italy: F. Sacchetto, 1871): 9. Interestingly, the copy of this book that I examined had been gifted to none other than Joseph Barnard Davis.

14. Cesare Lombroso and Gina Lombroso, *Criminal Man, According to the Classification of Cesare Lombroso* (New York: Putnam, 1911).

15. Charles K. Mills, "Presidential Address, Including Arrested and Aberrant Development of Fissures and Gyres in the Brains of Paranoiacs, Criminals, Idiots, and Negroes and Description of a Chinese Brain," *Journal of Nervous and Mental Disease* 13, nos. 9 and 10 (1886): 517–53.

16. Ilaria Natali, "Permeable Borders: Bram Stoker's Dracula and Its Sources," in I. Natali and A. Volpone (eds.), *"The Common Darkness Where the Dreams Abide": Perspectives on Irish Gothic and Beyond* (Perugia, Italy: Aguaplano Libri, 2018): 137–58.

17. Stephen Arata, "The Sedulous Ape: Atavism, Professionalism, and Stevenson's *Jekyll and Hyde*," *Fictions of Loss in the Victorian Fin De Siècle: Identity and Empire* (Cambridge, UK: Cambridge University Press, 1996).

18. Raymond B. Fosdick, "Passing of the Bertillon System of Identification," *Journal of Criminal Law and Criminology* 6, no. 3 (1915): 8; W. A. M'Corn, "Degeneration in Criminals as Shown by the Bertillon System of Measurement and Photographs," *American Journal of Insanity* 53 (July 1896): 47–56.

19. Austin Flint, "The Coming Role of the Medical Profession in the Scientific Treatment of Crime and Criminals," *New York Medical Journal* LXII (1895): 481–90; Thomas B. Keyes, "Criminality and Degeneracy; Its Treatment by Surgery and Hypnotism," *Medico-Legal Journal*, XV (1897–98): 366–74; Sophia McClelland, "Criminals the Product of Hereditary Degeneracy," *Medical Record* XLII (July 1892): 96–100; John Morris, "Crime; Its Physiology and Parthenogenesis: How Far Can Medical Men Aid in Its Prevention?" *Maryland Medical Journal* XX (April 1889): 501–12.

20. F. E. Daniel, "Should Insane Criminals or Sexual Perverts Be Allowed to Procreate?," *Medico-Legal Journal of New York* 11, no. 4 (1893): 272–92.

4. From Sir Francis Galton to Connecticut

1. Kostas Kampourakis, *How We Get Mendel Wrong, and Why It Matters: Challenging the Narrative of Mendelian Genetics* (New York: CRC Press, 2024).

2. Charles Darwin, *The Variation of Animals and Plants Under Domestication*, 2nd edition (London: John Murray, 1885).

3. Iris Sandler, "Pierre Louis Moreau De Maupertuis: A Precursor of Mendel?," *Journal of the History of Biology* 16, no. 1 (1983): 100–36.

4. Charles Darwin to T. H. Huxley, July 12, 1865, "Letter no. 4870," Darwin Correspondence Project, darwinproject.ac.uk/DCP-LETT-4870.xml. Accessed August 23, 2018.

5. Charles Darwin to Francis Galton, July 24, 1853, "Letter no. 1525," Darwin Correspondence Project, darwinproject.ac.uk/letter/?docId=letters/DCP-LETT-1525.xml. Accessed August 23, 2018.

6. Martin Brookes, *Extreme Measures: The Dark Visions and Bright Ideas of Francis Galton* (London: Bloomsbury, 2004).

7. Francis Galton, *Hereditary Genius: An Inquiry Into Its Laws and Consequences*, 2nd edition (London: Macmillan & Co., 1892). Galton actually coined the nature versus nurture dichotomy in his later book, *English Men of Science: Their Nature and Nurture* (London: Macmillan & Co., 1874).

8. Charles Darwin to Francis Galton, December 23, 1869, "Letter no. 7032," Darwin Correspondence Project, darwinproject.ac.uk/letter/?docId=letters/DCP-LETT-7032.xml. Accessed August 23, 2018.

9. Francis Galton, *Hereditary Genius*, op. cit.

10. Francis Galton to Charles Darwin, December 11, 1869, "Letter no. 7026," Darwin Correspondence Project, darwinproject.ac.uk/DCP-LETT-7026. Accessed August 25, 2018.

11. Francis Galton to Charles Darwin, April 9, 1871, "Letter no. 7671," Darwin Correspondence Project, darwinproject.ac.uk/DCP-LETT-7671. Accessed August 25, 2018.

12. Francis Galton, "Hereditary Improvement," *Fraser's Magazine* 7 (1873): 116–30.

13. Francis Galton, "Letter to the Editor," *The Times of London*, June 5, 1873, galton.org/letters/africa-for-chinese/AfricaForTheChinese.htm.

14. Francis Galton, "Eugenics: Its Definition, Scope, and Aims," *The American Journal of Sociology* 10, no. 1 (July 1904).

15. H. G. Wells, in Francis Galton, "Eugenics," op. cit.

16. Lucia L. Jaquith, "The Menace of the Feeble-Minded," *The American Journal of Nursing* 14, no. 4 (1914): 268–71.

17. Albert O. Wright, "The New Philanthropy," *Proceedings of the National Conference of Charities and Correction* 23 (1896).

18. Ibid.

19. Connecticut HB 681, Public Acts, January 1895, Session 667.

20. "Asexualization of Criminals and Degenerates," *Michigan Law Journal* 6, no. 12 (1897).

21. Ibid.

22. Ibid.

23. Ibid.

5. The Indiana Plan

1. Alfred C. Wood II, "The Results of Castration and Vasectomy in Hypertrophy of the Prostate Gland," *Annals of Surgery* 32, no. 3 (1900): 309–50.

2. A. J. Ochsner, "Surgical treatment of habitual criminals," *JAMA* 32, no. 16 (1899): 867–68.

3. Ibid.

4. See, for instance, William M. Kantor, "Beginnings of Sterilization in America," *Journal of Heredity* 28, no. 11 (1937): 374–76.

5. Ibid.

6. Angela Gugliotta, "'Dr. Sharp with His Little Knife': Therapeutic and Punitive Origins of Eugenic Vasectomy—Indiana, 1892–1921," *Journal of the History of Medicine and Allied Sciences* 53, no. 4 (1998): 371–406.

7. William M. Kantor, "Beginnings of Sterilization," op. cit.

6. The American Eugenics Triangle

1. See their exchanges January 2, 1902, to February 15, 1910, Davenport papers (via the American Philosophical Society, Philadelphia).

2. Daniel Kevles, *In the Name of Eugenics: Genetics and the Uses of Human Heredity* (New York: Knopf, 1985).

3. Charles Davenport, *Heredity in Relation to Eugenics* (New York: Henry Holt, 1911).

4. Lutz Kaelber, "Eugenics: Compulsory Sterilization in 50 American States," presentation at the 2012 Social Science History Association, University of Vermont, uvm.edu/%7Elkaelber/eugenics.

5. P. Laughlin et al., "Acquired or inherited? A eugenical comedy in four acts," performed at the Eugenics Records Office, Cold Spring Harbor, NY, August 4, 1913 (via the American Philosophical Society Archive, Philadelphia).

6. Harry Hamilton Haughlin, *Eugenical Sterilization in the United States* (Chicago: Psychopathic Laboratory of the Municipal Court of Chicago, 1922).

7. Sterilization data from Lutz Kaelber, "Eugenics," op. cit.

8. Howard Markel, "How Dr. Kellogg's World-Renowned Health Spa Made Him a Wellness Titan," *PBS NewsHour*, August 18, 2017, pbs.org/newshour/health/dr-kelloggs-world-renowned-health-spa-made-wellness-titan.

9. J. H. Kellogg, "Needed—a New Human Race," in *Proceedings of the First National Conference on Race Betterment, January 8, 9, 10, 11, 12, 1914, Battle Creek, Michigan* (Battle Creek, MI: Gage Printing Co., 1914).

10. Alexandra Minna Stern, *Eugenic Nation: Faults and Frontiers of Better Breeding in Modern America*, 2nd edition (Oakland: University of California Press, 2015).

11. Charles Davenport, "The Importance to the State of Eugenic Investigation," in *Proceedings of the First National Conference on Race Betterment*, op. cit.

12. Sterilization data from Lutz Kaelber, "Eugenics," op. cit.

13. F. O. Butler, "A Quarter of a Century's Experience in Sterilization of Mental Defectives in California," *American Journal of Mental Deficiency* 49, no.4 (1945); Phil Barber, "How Sonoma County Became the Center of America's Forced Sterilization Movement," *Santa Rosa Press Democrat*, November 4, 2021, pressdemocrat.com/article/news/how-sonoma-county-became-the-dark-center-of-americas-forced-sterilization.

14. Michael Hiltzik, "Caltech Faces Reckoning over Its Links to Eugenics and Sterilization Movement," *Los Angeles Times*, July 7, 2020, latimes.com/business/story/2020-07-07/caltech-robert-millikan-eugenics-sterilization.

15. "Table of sterilizations done in state institutions under state laws up to and including the year 1940," Harry H. Laughlin Papers, Truman State University (via Eugenics Archive, eugenicsarchive.org/html/eugenics/static/images/1199.html).

16. Paul R. Spitzzeri, "The Slippery Slope of Social Engineering: The Case of Paul B. Popenoe, 1915–1930," The Homestead Blog, February 28, 2020, homesteadmuseum.blog/2020/02/27/the-slippery-slope-of-social-engineering-the-case-of-paul-b-popenoe-1915-1930.

17. Paul Popenoe, "The German Sterilization Law," *Journal of Heredity* 25, no. 7 (1934): 257–60.

18. Paul Popenoe to E. S. Gosney (January 1926), Box 7, Folder 2, E. S. Gosney Papers & Human Betterment Foundation Archives, California Institute of Technology, Pasadena, CA.

19. Wendy Klein, "The Surprising History of Marriage Counseling," *American Experience*, PBS, October 19, 2018, pbs.org/wgbh/americanexperience/features/eugenics-surprising-history-of-marriage-counseling.

20. Paul Popenoe, *Problems of Human Reproduction* (Baltimore: Williams and Wilkins, 1926).

21. Paul Popenoe, *Modern Marriage—A Handbook* (New York: Macmillan, 1925).

22. George H. Beale, "First Clinic for Settling Home Trouble," *Whittier News*, February 6, 1930.

23. As well as their published works, see: "Data Summary—Insane Men and Women," Box 36, Folder 1, E. S. Gosney Papers & Human Betterment Foundation Archives, California Institute of Technology, Pasadena, CA; Alexandra Minna Stern, "Sterilized in the Name of Public Health: Race, Immigration, and Reproductive Control in Modern California," *American Journal of Public Health* 95, no. 7 (2005): 1128–38.

24. Jill Lepore, "Fixed," *The New Yorker*, March 22, 2010; "You Bet Your Life (TV Series 1950–1961) - Full Cast & Crew," IMDb, imdb.com/title/tt0042171/fullcredits.

25. Sara Boboltz, "Awful '50s Marriage Advice Shows What Our Mothers and Grandmothers Were Up Against," HuffPost, September 26, 2014, huffpost.com/entry/can-this-marriage-be-saved-advice_n_5829870.

7. Studying the Worst of Us

1. Brent Ruswick, "The Measure of Worthiness: The Rev. Oscar McCulloch and the Pauper Problem, 1877–1891," *Indiana Magazine of History* 104, no. 1 (2008): 3–35.

2. F. B. Sanborn (ed.), *Proceedings of the Seventh Annual National Conference of Charities and Correction* (Boston: A. Williams & Co., 1880).

3. Nicole Rafter (ed.), *White Trash: The Eugenic Family Studies, 1877–1919* (Boston: Northeastern University Press, 1988).

4. F. B. Sanborn, *Proceedings of the Seventh Annual National Conference*, op. cit.

5. Edward Morse Shepard, *The Work of a Social Teacher: Being a Memorial of Richard L. Dugdale* (New York: Society for Political Education, 1884).

6. Hamilton Cravens, *The Triumph of Evolution: Heredity Environment Controversy, 1900–1941* (Baltimore: Johns Hopkins University Press, 1998).

7. Elof Axel Carlson, "R. L. Dugdale and the Jukes Family: A Historical Injustice Corrected," *BioScience* 30, no. 8 (August 1980): 535–39.

8. Nicole Rafter, *White Trash*, op. cit.

8. Legal Scaffolding for Eugenics

1. *The State of Washington v. Peter Feilen*, 70 Wash. 65 (September 3, 1912).

2. Ibid.

3. *Davis v. Berry*, 216 F. 413, No. 9-A (United States District Court for the Southern District of Iowa, June 24, 1914).

4. Ibid.

5. *Smith v. Wayne Probate Judge*, 231 Mich. 409, No. 3 (Michigan Supreme Court, June 18, 1925).

6. Paul A. Lombardo, *Three Generations, No Imbeciles: Eugenics, the Supreme Court, and Buck v. Bell* (Baltimore: Johns Hopkins University Press, 2008).

7. *Buck v. Bell, Superintendent of State Colony for Epileptics and Feeble Minded*, 274 U.S. 200, No. 292 (Supreme Court of the United States, May 2, 1927).

8. Ibid.

9. Paul A. Lombardo, *Three Generations*, op. cit.

9. Drowning the "Great Race" Under a "Rising Tide of Color"

1. Joseph Jacobs, "On the Racial Characteristics of Modern Jews," *Journal of the Anthropological Institute of Great Britain and Ireland* 15 (1885): 54.

2. Benjamin Disraeli, *Tancred, or the New Crusade* (London: M. Walter Dunne, 1847).

3. Jonathan P. Spiro, "Patrician Racist: The Evolution of Madison Grant," PhD dissertation, University of California, Berkeley (2000).

4. Madison Grant, *The Passing of the Great Race; or, The Racial Basis of European History* (New York: Charles Scribner's Sons, 1916).

5. Lothrop Stoddard, *The Revolt Against Civilization: The Menace of the Under-Man* (New York: Charles Scribner's Sons, 1922): 239–42.

6. T. R. Ybarra, "Can White Races Be Submerged by Colored Hordes?," *The New York Times*, May 2, 1920.

7. Warren G. Harding, "Address of the President of the United States at the Celebration of the Semicentennial Founding of the City of Birmingham, Alabama," October 26, 1921, voicesofdemocracy.umd.edu/warren-g-harding-address-at-birmingham-speech-text.

8. F. Scott Fitzgerald, *The Great Gatsby* (New York: Charles Scribner's Sons, 1925).

10. A Global Eugenics Network

1. Antoine Prost, "War Losses," 1914-1918-Online, International Encyclopedia of the First World War, encyclopedia.1914-1918-online.net/article/war_losses.

2. Robert Wilson, "Eugenic family studies," Eugenics Archive, eugenicsarchive.ca/discover/encyclopedia/535eebbb7095aa0000000225, accessed September 5, 2024; and Nicole Rafter (ed.), *White Trash: The Eugenic Family Studies, 1877–1919* (Boston: Northeastern University Press, 1988).

3. "Exhibit of the Second International Congress of Eugenics," floor plans of exhibition hall, Second International Congress of Eugenics, Exhibits Book (via Eugenics Archive, eugenicsarchive.org/eugenics/image_header.pl?id=542&detailed=1).

4. Frank Gary Brooks, "Selling the Future Short," *Bios* 2, no. 3 (1931): 151–55.

5. Edwin Black, *War Against the Weak: Eugenics and America's Campaign to Create a Master Race* (New York: Dialog Press, 2012).

6. Ross Douthat, "Clarence Thomas's Dangerous Idea," *The New York Times*, June 1, 2019.

7. Edwin Black, *War Against the Weak*, op. cit.

8. Alexandra Minna Stern, "Gender and Sexuality: A Global Tour and Compass," in Alison Bashford and Philippa Levine (eds.), *The Oxford Handbook of the History of Eugenics* (New York: Oxford University Press, 2010).

9. *Actas de la II Conferencia Panamericana de Eugenesia y Homicultura de las Repúblicas Americanas* (Buenos Aires: Fascoli y Bindi, 1934).

10. Yolanda Eraso, "Biotypology, Endocrinology, and Sterilization: The Practice of Eugenics in the Treatment of Argentinian Women During the 1930s," *Bulletin of the History of Medicine* 81, no. 4 (2007): 793–822.

11. "The History—Northern Territory, 8. Bringing them home, Australian Human Rights Commission," humanrights.gov.au/our-work/bringing-them-home-8-history-northern-territory. Accessed September 5, 2024.

12. W. A. Plecker, "Virginia's Effort to Preserve Racial Integrity," in H. H. Laughlin et al. (eds.), *A Decade of Progress in Eugenics* (Baltimore: Williams & Wilkins, 1934).

13. Warwick Anderson, *The Cultivation of Whiteness: Science, Health, and Racial Destiny in Australia* (New York: Basic Books, 2003).

14. Cassia Roth, "The Degenerating Sex: Female Sterilisation, Medical Authority and Racial Purity in Catholic Brazil," *Medical History* 64, no. 2 (2020): 173–94.

15. Eugenics Archives (Canada), Social Sciences & Humanities Research Council of Canada (2010–2015), eugenicsarchive.ca.

16. W. E. Crusio, "*A Whisper Past: Childless after Eugenic Sterilization in Alberta*, by Leilani Muir," *Genes, Brain and Behavior* 14, no. 5 (2015): 439.

17. Leon Antonio Rocha, "Quentin Pan 潘光旦 in *The China Critic*," *China Heritage Quarterly* 30/31 (2012).

18. Yuehtsen J. Chung, "Eugenics in China and Hong Kong: Nationalism and Colonialism, 1890s–1940s," in A. Bashford and P. Levine (eds.), *The Oxford Handbook of the History of Eugenics* (New York: Oxford University Press, 2010).

19. Daniel S. Gewirtz, "Toward a Quality Population: China's Eugenic Sterilization of the Mentally Retarded," *NYLS Journal of International and Comparative Law* 15, no. 1 (1994): Article 6.

20. Sumiko Otsubo, "Between Two Worlds: Yamanouchi Shigeo and Eugenics in Early Twentieth-Century Japan," *Annals of Science* 62, no. 2 (2005): 205–31.

21. Quoted in Jennifer Robertson, "Blood Talks: Eugenic Modernity and the Creation of New Japanese," *History and Anthropology* 13, no. 3 (2002): 191–216.

22. Takashi Tsuchiya, "Eugenic Sterilizations in Japan and Recent Demands for Apology: A Report," *Newsletter of the Network on Ethics and Intellectual Disability* 3, no. 1 (1997): 1–4.

23. Siri Haavie, "Sterilization in Norway—A Dark Chapter?" *Eurozine*, April 9, 2003, eurozine.com/sterilization-in-norway-a-dark-chapter.

24. Dan Balz, "Sweden Sterilized Thousands of 'Useless' Citizens for Decades," *The Washington Post*, August 29, 1997; and G. Broberg and N. Roll-Hansen (eds.), *Eugenics and the Welfare State: Sterilization Policy in Denmark, Sweden, Norway, and Finland* (East Lansing: Michigan State University Press, 1996).

25. Martin Ericsson, "What happened to 'race' in race biology? The Swedish State Institute for Race Biology, 1936–1960," *Scandinavian Journal of History* 46 (2020): 125–48.

26. Regina Wecker. "Eugenics in Switzerland before and after 1945—a Continuum?," *Journal of Modern European History* 10, no. 4 (2012): 519–39.

27. Elizabeth Ortega et al., "Eugenics and Medicalization of Crime at the Early 20th Century in Uruguay," *Saúde e Sociedade* 27, no. 2 (2018): 354–66.

28. Nancy Stepan, "*The Hour of Eugenics*": Race, Gender, and Nation in Latin America (Ithaca, NY: Cornell University Press, 1991).

11. Making America White Again

1. *Grays Harbor Washingtonian* (June 14, 1934), cited in Alfred J. Hillier, "Albert Johnson, Congressman," *Pacific Northwest Quarterly* 36, no. 3 (1945): 195.

2. David Cahn, "The 1907 Bellingham Riots in Historical Context," The Seattle Civil Rights and Labor History Project, University of Washington, depts. washington.edu/civilr/bham_history.htm; Trevor Griffey, "Citizen Klan: Electoral Politics and the KKK in WA," The Seattle Civil Rights and Labor History Project, University of Washington, depts.washington.edu/civilr/kkk_politicians.htm; and "Jap Influx is Predicted," *San Pedro Daily News* 5, no. 312 (1907).

3. "KU KLUX KLAN: Washington Splurge," *Time* magazine, September 20, 1926.

4. Albert Johnson, speech before the House of Representatives, curiosity. lib.harvard.edu/immigration-to-the-united-states-1789-1930/catalog/39-990099887160203941.

5. Donald Trump, the Republican presidential candidate, spoke these words in the 2016 campaign: Jenna Johnson, "Trump Calls for 'Total and Complete Shutdown of Muslims Entering the United States,'" *The Washington Post*, December 7, 2015. Surely, the cheers from the white crowd were just as loud.

6. "Immigration Act of 1921 Imposes Quota System, 1921–1924," *Gale U.S. History In Context*, 2012, www.dentonisd.org/cms/lib/TX21000245/Centricity/Domain/535/Immigration%20Act.pdf.

7. Edwin Black, "Eugenics and the Nazis—the California connection," *SFGate*, November 9, 2003.

8. Adam Serwer, "Jeff Sessions's Unqualified Praise for a 1924 Immigration Law," *The Atlantic*, January 10, 2017.

9. See "Quotas by country under successive laws," in "Immigration Act of 1924," Wikipedia, wikipedia.org/w/index.php?title=Immigration_Act_of_1924&oldid=1089437804.

12. Nazi Ties

1. Godwin's Law is the humorous, somewhat exasperated insight that as any debate (especially online) increases in duration, the probability that someone will compare someone or something to Hitler or the Third Reich increases to near certainty. "Godwin's Law, n.," OED Online, Oxford University Press, oed.com/view/Entry/340583. Accessed January 2018.

2. Joseph L. Graves Jr., *The Emperor's New Clothes: Biological Theories of Race at the Millennium* (New Brunswick, NJ: Rutgers University Press, 2001).

3. Peter Campbell, "The 'Black Horror on the Rhine': Idealism, Pacifism, and Racism in Feminism and the Left in the Aftermath of the First World War," *Social History* 47 (2014): 471–96.

4. Stefan Kühl, *For the Betterment of the Race: The Rise and Fall of the International Movement for Eugenics and Racial Hygiene*, trans. L. Schofer (New York: Palgrave Macmillan, 2013).

5. Iris Wigger, "'Black Shame'—the campaign against 'racial degeneration' and female degradation in interwar Europe," *Race and Class* 51 (2010).

6. Stefan Kühl, *For the Betterment of the Race*, op. cit.

7. Robert Proctor, *Racial Hygiene: Medicine Under the Nazis* (Cambridge, MA: Harvard University Press, 1988): 344.

8. Peter Lehmann, "'Progressive' Psychiatry: Publisher J. F. Lehmann as Promoter of Social Psychiatry under Fascism," *Changes – An International Journal of Psychology and Psychotherapy* (England) 12, no. 1 (1994): 37–49.

9. D. Olusoga and C. W. Ericksen, *The Kaiser's Holocaust: Germany's Forgotten Genocide and the Colonial Roots of Nazism* (New York: Faber & Faber, 2011).

10. Erna Kurbegovic and Colette Leung, "Fischer, Eugen" (via Eugenics Archive, eugenicsarchive.ca/discover/connections/5233d0235c2ec500000000b0). Accessed March 28, 2018.

11. Hans Harmsen, "Berichte. Der international Kongreß für Bevölkerungswissenschaft und der Internationale Strafrechtskongreß," *Archiv für Bevölkerungswissenshaft und Bevölkerungspolitik* 5 (1935): 355–68.

13. To Murder Six Million

1. *Erbkrank* (1936), produced by Rassenpolitisches Amt der NSDAP, archive.org/details/1936-Rassenpolitisches-Amt-der-NSDAP-Erbkrank.

2. Stefan Kühl, *For the Betterment of the Race: The Rise and Fall of the International Movement for Eugenics and Racial Hygiene*, trans. L. Schofer (New York: Palgrave Macmillan, 2013).

3. James Q. Whitman, *Hitler's American Model: The United States and the Making of Nazi Race Law* (Princeton, NJ: Princeton University Press, 2017).

4. Chrisanne Beckner, "Darkness on the edge of campus: University's philanthropic 'godfather' was mad about eugenics," *Sacramento News & Review*, February 19, 2004.

5. Judy Scales-Trent, "Racial Purity Laws in the United States and Nazi Germany: The Targeting Process," *Human Rights Quarterly* 23, no. 2 (2001): 260–307.

6. Stefan Kühl, *The Nazi Connection: Eugenics, American Racism, and German National Socialism* (New York: Oxford University Press, 2001).

7. Robert Proctor, *Racial Hygiene: Medicine under the Nazis* (Cambridge, MA: Harvard University Press, 1988).

8. Quoted in Stefan Kühl, *For the Betterment of the Race*, op. cit.

9. Lothrop Stoddard, *Into the Darkness: Nazi Germany Today* (New York: Duell, Sloan & Pearce, 1940).

10. Robert J. Lifton, *The Nazi Doctors: Medical Killing and the Psychology of Genocide* (New York: Basic Books, 2000).

11. "The Moscow Conference; October 1943," The Avalon Project: Documents in Law, History and Diplomacy, Lillian Goldman Law Library, Yale Law School, avalon.law.yale.edu/wwii/moscow.asp.

12. Kevin Jon Heller, *The Nuremberg Military Tribunals and the Origins of International Criminal Law* (Oxford, UK: Oxford University Press, 2011).

13. Though it is true he was examined and fined by the US Army Counter Intelligence Corps and the "Office for War Crimes," Verschuer avoided a formal trial and received an appointment to the University of Münster, where he would later become dean. Sheila Faith Weiss, "After the Fall. Political Whitewashing, Professional Posturing, and personal Refashioning in the Postwar Career of Otmar Freiherr von Verschuer," *Isis* 101 (2010): 729–30.

14. Ibid.

15. Edwin Black, "Eugenics and the Nazis—the California connection," *SFGate*, November 9, 2003.

16. Gavin Schaffer, "'Scientific' Racism Again?: Reginald Gates, the *Mankind Quarterly* and the Question of 'Race' in Science after the Second World War," *Journal of American Studies* 41, no. 2 (2007): 253–78.

14. Puerto Rico: A Surplus Colonial Population

1. Pedro Ortiz, "The Tropics from a Public Health Standpoint," *Porto Rico Health Review* 11, no. 12 (1927): 3–13.

2. Lt. Col. Esteban Jimenez, Letter to the Editor: "Winship's Record in Puerto Rico Was Hardly Heroic," *Puerto Rico Herald*, May 24, 2004.

3. A. W. Maldonado, *Luis Muñoz Marín: Puerto Rico's Democratic Revolution* (San Juan: Editorial Universidad de Puerto Rico, 2006).

4. "Sterilization Study Is Urged by Winship," *The New York Times*, February 10, 1937.

5. Annette B. Ramírez de Arellano and Conrad Seipp, *Colonialism, Catholicism and Contraception: A History of Birth Control in Puerto Rico* (Chapel Hill: University of North Carolina Press, 2014).

6. Kurt W. Back et al., "Population Control in Puerto Rico: The Formal and Informal Framework," *Law and Contemporary Problems* 25, no. 3 (1960): 558–76.

7. J. Mayone Stycos, "Female Sterilization in Puerto Rico," *Eugenics Quarterly* 1, no. 1 (1954): 3–8.

8. Bonnie Mass, "Puerto Rico: A Case Study of Population Control," *Latin American Perspectives* 4, no. 4 (1977): 66–81.

9. Laura Briggs, *Reproducing Empire: Race, Sex, Science, and U.S. Imperialism in Puerto Rico* (Berkeley: University of California Press, 2002).

10. *La Operación* (1982), directed by Ana María García, youtu.be/uoJoWMbRxvM.

11. Drew C. Pendergrass and Michelle Y. Raji, "The Bitter Pill: Harvard and the Dark History of Birth Control," *Harvard Crimson*, September 28, 2017.

12. Harriet B. Presser, *Sterilization and Fertility Decline in Puerto Rico*, Population Monograph Series 13 (Berkeley: University of California Press, 1973).

13. Helen Rodriquez-Trias, "The Women's Health Movement: Women Take Power," in V. Sidel and R. Sidel (eds.), *Reforming Medicine: Lessons of the Last Quarter Century* (New York: Pantheon, 1984).

14. McCormick to Sanger, May 31, 1955, cited in Lara Marks, "'A "Cage" of Ovulating Females': The History of the Early Oral Contraceptive Pill Clinical Trials, 1950–1959," in S. de Chadarevian and H. Kamminga (eds.), *Molecularizing Biology and Medicine: New Practices and Alliances, 1920s to 1970s* (London: Taylor & Francis, 1998).

15. Drew C. Pendergrass and Michelle Y. Raji, "The Bitter Pill," op. cit.

16. McCormick to Sanger, op. cit.

17. Nick Thimmesch, "Puerto Rico and Birth Control," *Journal of Marriage and Family* 30, no. 2 (1968): 252–62.

18. See, for example, Marc Dhont, "History of oral contraception," *European Journal of Contraception & Reproductive Health Care* 15, Suppl. 2 (2010): S12–S18.

19. Theresa Vargas, "Guinea Pigs or Pioneers? How Puerto Rican Women Were Used to Test the Birth Control Pill," *The Washington Post*, October 28, 2021.

20. Katherine Brind'Amour and Benjamin Garcia, "*Humanae Vitae* (1968), by Pope Paul VI," Embryo Project Encyclopedia, November 13, 2007, embryo.asu.edu/pages/humanae-vitae-1968-pope-paul-vi.

21. Lara Marks, "Human Guinea Pigs? The History of the Early Oral Contraceptive Clinical Trials." *History and Technology* 15 (1999): 263–88.

22. Laura Briggs, *Reproducing Empire*, op. cit.

23. Harriet B. Presser, "Puerto Rico: Recent Trends in Fertility and Sterilization," *Family Planning Perspectives* 12, no. 2 (1980): 102–6.

24. Drew C. Pendergrass and Michelle Y. Raji, "The Bitter Pill," op. cit.

15. The Population Control Industrial Complex

1. Ian Dowbiggin, *The Sterilization Movement and Global Fertility in the Twentieth Century* (New York: Oxford University Press, 2008).

2. "Composite Report of the President's Committee to Study the United States Military Assistance Program" (August 17, 1959), https://edocs.nps.edu/2012/December/pcaaa444.pdf.

3. "Letter of Draper Committee on Foreign Aid," *The New York Times*, July 24, 1959.

4. Betsy Hartmann, "Population Control I: Birth of an Ideology," *International Journal of Health Services: Planning, Administraion, Evaluation* 27, no. 3 (1997): 523–40.

5. John W. Finney, "Eisenhower Backs Birth Curb Study," *The New York Times*, June 23, 1965.

6. Arthur R. Jensen, "How much can we boost IQ and scholastic achievement?," *Harvard Educational Review* 39, no. 1 (1969): 1–123.

7. Angela Saini, "Draper's Millions: The Philanthropic Wellspring of Modern Race Science," Undark, December 16, 2022, race.undark.org/articles/drapers-millions-the-philanthropic-wellspring-of-modern-race-science.

8. "Letter by Eisenhower on Birth Control," *The New York Times*, June 23, 1965.

9. Marc Dhont, "History of Oral Contraception," *European Journal of Contraception & Reproductive Health Care* 15, Suppl. 2 (2010): S12–S18.

10. *Time* magazine, November 27, 1964, cover, content.time.com/time/magazine/0,9263,7601641127,00.html; and the Hugh Moore Fund Collection, Public Policy Papers, Department of Special Collections, Princeton University Library, arks.princeton.edu/ark:/88435/12579s25h.

11. Laura Briggs, *Reproducing Empire: Race, Sex, Science, and U.S. Imperialism in Puerto Rico* (Berkeley: University of California Press, 2002).

12. Betsy Hartmann, "Population Control II: The Population Establishment Today," *International Journal of Health Services* 27, no. 3 (1997): 541–57.

13. Richard Nixon, "Special Message to the Congress on Problems of Population Growth," The American Presidency Project, presidency.ucsb.edu/node/239625.

14. Johanna Schoen, *Choice and Coercion: Birth Control, Sterilization, and Abortion in Public Health and Welfare* (Chapel Hill: University of North Carolina Press, 2005).

16. The Population Bomb Bomb

1. Jonathan P. Spiro, "Patrician Racist: The Evolution of Madison Grant," PhD dissertation, University of California, Berkeley, 2000.

2. Bonnie Mass, "An Historical Sketch of the American Population Control Movement," *International Journal of Health Services* 4, no. 4 (1974): 651–76.

3. Aditi Kharod, "A 1960s Population Control Organization Rebranded in 2002. Now It's Recruiting UNC Students," NC Newsline, November 20, 2019, ncnewsline.com/2019/11/20/a-1960s-population-control-organization-rebranded-in-2002-now-its-recruiting-unc-students.

4. Charles C. Mann, "The Book That Incited a Worldwide Fear of Overpopulation," *Smithsonian* magazine, January 2018.

5. Paul R. Ehrlich, with Anne H. Ehrlich, *The Population Bomb* (New York: Sierra Club/Ballantine Books,1968).

6. Ibid.

7. "WOI-TV Interviews Dr. Paul Ehrlich (April 24, 1970)," Iowa State University, Special Collections and University Archives, youtu.be/YZWiRaIkXxg.

8. Stewart Brand, *Whole Earth Discipline: An Ecopragmatist Manifesto* (New York: Viking Penguin, 2009).

9. Ben Wattenberg, "The Nonsense Explosion," American Enterprise Institute, August 26, 2013, aei.org/articles/aei-classics-the-nonsense-explosion.

10. "Family Planning (1968)," produced by Walt Disney Productions for the Population Council, youtu.be/t2DkiceqmzU.

11. "The Tonight Show Starring Johnny Carson (aired January 31, 1980), Dr. Paul Ehrlich," youtu.be/6E5lUNBk3zQ?si=cUtB-QXhDoH1dd4I.

12. M. F. Franda, "The World Population Conference: an international extravaganza," *Southeast Europe* 21, no. 2 (1974): 1–9.

13. Hannah Ritchie et al., "Population Growth," Our World in Data, https://ourworldindata.org/population-growth.

14. Matthew Connelly, *Fatal Misconception: The Struggle to Control World Population* (Cambridge, MA: Harvard University Press, 2008).

15. Betsy Hartmann, *Reproductive Rights and Wrongs: The Global Politics of Population Control*, 3rd edition (Chicago: Haymarket Books, 2016).

17. Emergencies

1. Paul R. Ehrlich, with Anne H. Ehrlich, *The Population Bomb* (New York: Sierra Club/Ballantine Books, 1968).

2. Lyndon B. Johnson, "Address in San Francisco at the 20th Anniversary Commemorative Session of the United Nations," The American Presidency Project, presidency.ucsb.edu/node/241692.

3. Charles C. Mann, "The Book That Incited a Worldwide Fear of Overpopulation," *Smithsonian* magazine, January 2018.

4. Kathleen D. McCarthy, "From government to grass-roots reform: the Ford Foundation's population programmes in South Asia, 1959–1981," *Voluntas* 6, no. 3 (1995): 298.

5. Robert Zubrin, "The Population Control Holocaust," *The New Atlantis* 35 (2012).

6. Dylan Matthews and Byrd Pinkerton, "'The Time of Vasectomy': How American Foundations Fueled a Terrible Atrocity in India," Vox, June 5, 2019, vox.com/future-perfect/2019/6/5/18629801/emergency-in-india-1975-indira-gandhi-sterilization-ford-foundation.

7. *Population and the American Future: The Report of the Commission on Population Growth and the American Future* (New York: Signet, 1972).

8. Stephen Mosher, *Population Control: Real Costs, Illusory Benefits* (New York: Routledge, 2008).

9. NSC Under-Secretaries Committee, "First Annual Report on U.S. International Population Policy," July 29, 1976; in *Foreign Relations of the United States, 1969–1976, Volume E–14, Part 1, Documents on the United Nations, 1973–1976*, Department of State, Office of the Historian, history.state.gov/historicaldocuments/frus1969-76ve14p1/d125.

10. Anuradha Mascarenhas, "All They Wanted Were Men. Any Man," *Indian Express*, July 5, 2015.

11. Hannah Green, "The Legacy of India's Quest to Sterilize Millions of Men," Pulitzer Center, October 1, 2018, pulitzercenter.org/stories/legacy-indias-quest-sterilize-millions-men.

12. Anuradha Mascarenhas, "All They Wanted Were Men," op. cit.

13. NSC Under-Secretaries Committee, "First Annual Report," op. cit.

14. Robert S. McNamara, "McNamara on Population Growth: The 1980s and Beyond," *Population and Development Review* 5, no. 4 (1979): 736–39.

15. T. K. Sundari Ravindran, "Women and the Politics of Population and Development in India," *Reproductive Health Matters* 1, no. 1 (1993): 26–38.

16. "India Sterilisations: More Chhattisgarh Botched Cases," BBC News, November 12, 2014, bbc.com/news/world-asia-india-30024588.

17. H. S. D. Cole et al. (eds.), *Models of Doom: A Critique of* The Limits to Growth (New York: Universal Books, 1973).

18. Aileen Clarke, "See How the One-Child Policy Changed China," *National Geographic*, November 13, 2015.

19. Andrew Mullen, "What Was China's One-Child Policy and Why Was It So Controversial?," *South China Morning Post*, June 1, 2021.

20. Yuehtsen Juliette Chung, "The Postwar Return of Eugenics and the Dialectics of Scientific Practice in China," *Middle Ground Journal* 3 (2011): 1–50.

21. Emily Feng, "China's Former 1-Child Policy Continues to Haunt Families," NPR, July 4, 2021, npr.org/2021/06/21/1008656293/the-legacy-of-the-lasting-effects-of-chinas-1-child-policy.

22. Steven Mufson, "China Softens Bill on Eugenics," *The Washington Post*, December 30, 1993.

23. "China Cuts Uighur Births with IUDs, Abortion, Sterilization," AP News, April 20, 2021, apnews.com/article/ap-top-news-international-news-weekend-reads-china-health-269b3de1af34e17c1941a514f78d764c.

24. Conor Finnegan, "China Conducting Mass Sterilization on Muslim Minorities That Could Amount to Genocide: Report," ABC News, June 29, 2020, abcnews.go.com/Politics/china-conducting-mass-sterilization-muslim-minorities-amount-genocide/story?id=71519132.

25. Jelke Boesten, "Free Choice or Poverty Alleviation? Population Politics in Peru under Alberto Fujimori," *European Review of Latin American and Caribbean Studies* 82 (April 2007): 3–20.

26. Alicia Ely Yamin, "In Memoriam: Giulia Tamayo, 1958–2014," *Health and Human Rights Journal* 16, no. 2 (2014).

27. "The Quipo Project," Chaka Studio, interactive.quipu-project.com/#/en/quipu/intro.

28. Jacquelyn Kovarik, "Why Don't We Talk About Peru's Forced Sterilizations?," *The New Republic*, October 8, 2018; and Leila Miller, "Tied down and Sterilized: Peru's Dark History of Family Planning," *Los Angeles Times*, October 29, 2019.

29. "A Public Talk by Keiko Fujimori," Weatherhead Center for International Affairs, Harvard University, September 30, 2015, wcfia.harvard.edu/event/special-event-09-30-15.

18. Resistance, Weak and Strong

1. Roy Reed, "'Bloody Sunday' Was Year Ago," *The New York Times*, March 6, 1966.

2. Aniko Bodroghkozy, "How the images of John Lewis being beaten during 'Bloody Sunday' went viral," The Conversation, July 23, 2020, theconversation.com/how-the-images-of-john-lewis-being-beaten-during-bloody-sunday-went-viral-143080.

3. Elazar Barkan, *The Retreat of Scientific Racism: Changing Concepts of Race in Britain and the United States between the World Wars* (Cambridge, UK: Cambridge University Press, 1993).

4. Robin Marantz Henig, "The Life and Legacy of Paul de Kruif," The Alicia Patterson Foundation, 2002, aliciapatterson.org/stories/life-and-legacy-paul-de-kruif; Clarence Darrow, "The Eugenics Cult," *American Mercury* 8 (1926): 129–37; see also Darrow, "The Edwardses and the Jukeses," *American Mercury* 6 (1925): 147–57.

5. *Hearing before the House Committee on Immigration and Naturalization*, 68th Cong., 1st Sess. (Washington: Government Printing Office, 1924): 512; and Kenneth M. Ludmerer, *Genetics and the American Society: A Historical Appraisal* (Baltimore: Johns Hopkins University Press, 1972).

6. Elazar Barkan, "Reevaluating Progressive Eugenics: Herbert Spencer Jennings and the 1924 Immigration Legislation," *Journal of the History of Biology* 24, no. 1 (1991): 91–112.

7. Raymond Pearl, "Breeding Better Men: The New Science of Eugenics Which Would Elevate the Race by Producing Higher Types," *The World's Work* 19, no. 8 (1908): 9818–24.

8. Raymond Pearl, "The Biology of Superiority." *American Mercury*, November 12, 1927.

9. Bentley Glass and Curt Stern, "Geneticists Embattled: Their Stand against Rampant Eugenics and Racism in America during the 1920s and 1930s," *Proceedings of the American Philosophical Society* 130, no. 1 (1986): 130–54; and Melissa Hendricks, "Raymond Pearl's 'Mingled Mess,'" *Johns Hopkins Magazine*, April 2006, pages.jh.edu/jhumag/0406web/pearl.html.

10. Elazar Barkan, *The Retreat of Scientific Racism: Changing Concepts of Race in Britain and the United States between the World Wars* (Cambridge, UK: Cambridge University Press, 1992).

11. Stephen J. Gould, *The Mismeasure of Man* (New York: W. W. Norton, 1996).

12. See, for instance, John Lewis, "Mississippi's 'Genocide' Bill," *The Gazette and Daily*, June 8, 1964, newspapers.com/clip/19898004/mississippi-sterilization-1964.

13. As quoted in the Student Nonviolent Coordinating Committee pamphlet, "Genocide in Mississippi," 1964; see Tulane University Digital Library, digitallibrary.tulane.edu/islandora/object/tulane%3A21196.

14. Julius Paul, "State Eugenic Sterilization Laws in American Thought and Practice," unpublished manuscript (Walter Reed Army Institute of Research, 1965).

15. Keisha N. Blain, "Fannie Lou Hamer Sounded the Alarm on Forced Sterilization," Bitch Media, October 5, 2020, bitchmedia.org/article/fannie-lou-hamer-keisha-blain-excerpt.

16. Ibid.

17. "Fannie Lou Hamer," *American Experience*, PBS/WGBH, April 24, 2014, pbs. org/wgbh/americanexperience/features/freedomsummer-hamer.

18. Victoria F. Nourse, *In Reckless Hands:* Skinner v. Oklahoma *and the Near-Triumph of American Eugenics* (New York: W. W. Norton, 2008).

19. Julius Paul, "State Eugenic Sterilization Laws in American Thought and Practice," op. cit.

20. Lutz Kaelber, "Eugenics: Compulsory Sterilization in 50 American States," presentation at the 2012 Social Science History Association, Department of Sociology, University of Vermont, uvm.edu/%7Elkaelber/eugenics/OK/OK.html.

19. From Population Control to Poverty Control

1. Martha J. Bailey, "Reexamining the Impact of Family Planning Programs on US Fertility: Evidence from the War on Poverty and the Early Years of Title X," *American Economic Journal: Applied Economics*, 4, no. 2 (2012): 62–97.

2. Julius Paul, "State Eugenic Sterilization Laws in American Thought and Practice," unpublished manuscript (Walter Reed Army Institute of Research, 1965); Paul cites Richard Hofstadter, "The Pseudo-Conservative Revolt," in Daniel Bell (ed.), *The Radical Right* (Garden City, NY: Doubleday, 1964).

3. William Green, "The Odyssey of Depo-Provera: Contraceptives, Carcinogenic Drugs, and Risk-Management Analyses," *Food, Drug, Cosmetic Law Journal* 42, no. 4 (1987): 567–87.

4. "Clinic Defends Sterilization of 2 Girls, 12 and 14," *The New York Times*, June 28, 1973.

5. *Relf v. Weinberger*, No. Civ. A. Nos. 73-1557 (Consolidated with 74-243; US District Court for District of Columbia, July 17, 1973).

6. Dorothy E. Roberts, *Killing the Black Body: Race, Reproduction, and the Meaning of Liberty*, Twentieth Anniversary Edition (New York: Vintage, 2014).

7. Gregory M. Dorr, "Protection or Control? Women's Health, Sterilization Abuse, and *Relf v. Weinberger*," in P. Lombardo (ed.), *A Century of Eugenics in America: From the Indiana Experiment to the Human Genome Era* (Bloomington: Indiana University Press, 2011).

8. "Sterilized: Why?," *Time* magazine, July 23, 1973.

9. "The Belmont Report," Office for Human Research Protections, US Department of Health and Human Services, April 18, 1979, hhs.gov/ohrp/regulations-and-policy/belmont-report/read-the-belmont-report/index.html.

10. Alexandra Minna Stern, "STERILIZED in the Name of Public Health," *American Journal of Public Health* 95, no. 7 (2005): 1128–38.

11. Elena R. Gutiérrez, "Policing Pregnant Pilgrims: Situating the Sterilization Abuse of Mexican-Origin Women in Los Angeles County," in Georgina Feldberg et al. (eds.), *Women, Heath, and Nation: Canada and the United States since 1945* (Montreal: McGill-Queen's University Press, 2003).

12. *A Health Research Group Study on Surgical Sterilization: Present Abuses and Proposed Regulations* (Washington, DC: Health Research Group, 1973); and Nicole L. Novak and Natalie Lira, "California Once Targeted Latinas for Forced Sterilization," *Smithsonian* magazine, March 22, 2018.

13. Marcela Valdes, "When Doctors Took 'Family Planning' Into Their Own Hands," *The New York Times Magazine*, February 1, 2016.

14. Maya Manian, "The Story of *Madrigal v. Quilligan*: Coerced Sterilization of Mexican-American Women," University of San Francisco Law Research Paper No. 2018-04.

15. Alexandra Minna Stern, "STERILIZED in the Name of Public Health," op. cit.

16. Maya Manian, "The Story of *Madrigal v. Quilligan*," op. cit.

17. *Akwesasne Notes* 7, no. 3 (1974): 8 (via American Indian Digital History Project, aidhp.com/items/show/35).

18. Jane Lawrence, "The Indian Health Service and the Sterilization of Native American Women," *American Indian Quarterly* 24, no. 3 (2000): 400–19.

19. Robert E. McGarrah, "Voluntary Female Sterilization: Abuses, Risks and Guidelines," *Hastings Center Report* 4, no. 3 (1974): 5–7.

20. Claudia Dreifus, "Sterilizing the Poor," *The Progressive* 39 (1975): 13, 15–17.

21. Suzanne Tessler, "Compulsory Sterilization Practices," *Frontiers: A Journal of Women Studies* 1, no. 2 (1976): 52–66.

22. Jane Lawrence, "The Indian Health Service and the Sterilization of Native American Women," op cit.

23. Russell R. de Alvarez, MD (moderator), "Panel Discussion on Contraception & Sterilization," *American Journal of Obstetrics & Gynecology* 89, 3 (1964): 392–94.

24. John Mohawk, "Native People and the Right to Survive," *Akwesasne Notes* 11, no. 2 (1979): 4 (via American Indian Digital History Project, aidhp.com/items/show/54).

25. Myla Vicenti Carpio, "The Lost Generation: American Indian Women and Sterilization Abuse," *Social Justice* 31, no. 4 (2004): 42.

26. Quoted in Brooke Hadley, "The Sterilization of Native American Women in Oklahoma," Master of Arts thesis, University of Oklahoma, 2021.

27. "Indians and Medicine: Sterilization and Genocide—Dr. Connie Uri," KPFK, September 25, 1974, pacificaradioarchives.org/recording/bc1963.

28. "Indians face 'cultural genocide' threats," *Daily Herald*, May 23, 1977.

29. Brooke Hadley, "Sterilization of Native American Women in Oklahoma," op. cit.

30. "Investigation of Allegations Concerning Indian Health Service," US Government Accountability Office, November 4, 1976, gao.gov/products/hrd-77-3.

31. Ibid.

32. Jane Lawrence, "The Indian Health Service and the Sterilization of Native American Women," op. cit.

33. "About Us," Indian Health Service, Office of Urban Indian Health Programs, ihs.gov/urban/aboutus. Accessed March 13, 2022.

34. "Brief History of the Indian Health Care Improvement Act," National Indian Health Board, Tribal Health Reform Resource Center, nihb.org/tribalhealthreform/ihcia-history. Accessed March 13, 2022.

35. Kathryn Krase, "Sterilization Abuse: The Policies Behind the Practice," *National Women's Health Network Newsletter*, January 5, 1996; republished as "The Politics of Women's Health: Sterilization Abuse," by Our Bodies Ourselves Health Resource Center, ourbodiesourblog.org/book/companion-id-31-compID-55.html.

36. For instance, Garland E. Allen, "A History of Eugenics in the Class Struggle," *Science for the People* 6, no. 2 (1974).

37. Eric Eyre, "W.Va. House passes repeal of forced sterilization law," *Charleston Gazette-Mail*, March 25, 2013.

38. Philip R. Reilly, *The Surgical Solution: A History of Involuntary Sterilization in the United States* (Baltimore: Johns Hopkins University Press, 1991).

39. D'Vera Cohn, "Five States Have Cut Welfare Benefits below 1980 Levels," United Press International, November 2, 1981.

40. Mary Lenz, "A Poll on Killing and Sterilizing," *The Texas Observer*, March 20, 1981.

41. "Sequels," *The Texas Observer*, April 3, 1981.

42. George Gallup, "Illegitimacy Support Opposed by Majority," *The Washington Post*, January 27, 1965.

20. Sterilizing Criminals Again

1. Mary A. Telfer et al., "YY Syndrome in an American Negro," *The Lancet* 291, no. 7533 (1968): 95; and Mary A. Telfer et al., "Incidence of Gross Chromosomal Errors among Tall Criminal American Males," *Science* 159, no. 3820 (1968): 1249–50.

2. E. A. Whitney and M. M. Schick, "Some Results of Selective Sterilization," *Proceedings and Addresses of the 55th Annual Session of the American Association on Mental Deficiency* (1931): 332–33.

3. Patricia Jacobs et al., "Aggressive Behaviour, Mental Sub-normality and the XYY Male," *Nature* 208 (1965): 1351–52.

4. "Getty tells Speck case plea basis; 10 issues are raised regarding trial," *Chicago Tribune*, November 26, 1968.

5. "Of chromosomes & crime," *Time* magazine, May 3, 1968; "Born bad?" *Newsweek*, May 6, 1968; Stuart Auerbach, "Genetic abnormality is basis for acquittal," *The Washington Post*, October 10, 1968; Lloyd Garrison, "French murder jury rejects chromosome defect as defense," *The New York Times*, October 15, 1968; and "Criminal law: Question of Y," *Time* magazine, October 25, 1968.

6. Matt Roush, "Critic's corner," *USA Today*, November 17, 1993; and David Hochman, "Horatio hunts a natural-born killer," *TV Guide*, May 7–13, 2007.

7. "Alien 3," IMDb, imdb.com/title/tt0103644.

8. Clyde Haberman, "When Youth Violence Spurred 'Superpredator' Fear," *The New York Times*, April 6, 2014.

9. Robert Mackey and Zaid Jilani, "Hillary Clinton Still Haunted by Discredited Rhetoric on 'Superpredators,'" The Intercept, February 25, 2016, theintercept.com/2016/02/25/activists-want-hillary-clinton-apologize-hyping-myth-superpredators-1996.

10. Christine Samanns et al., "Gene for non-specific X-linked mental retardation maps in the pericentromeric region," *American Journal of Medical Genetics* 38, nos. 2–3 (1991): 224–27; and H. G. Brunner et al., "Abnormal behavior associated with a point mutation in the structural gene for monoamine oxidase A," *Science* 262, no. 5133 (1993): 578–80.

11. Ann Gibbons, "Tracking the Evolutionary History of a 'Warrior' Gene," *Science* 304, no. 5672 (2004): 818.

12. John Horgan, "Code Rage: The 'Warrior Gene' Makes Me Mad! (Whether I Have It or Not)," *Scientific American* Blog Network, April 26, 2011, blogs. scientificamerican.com/cross-check/code-rage-the-warrior-gene-makes-me-mad-whether-i-have-it-or-not.

13. Carroll Bogert and Lynnell Hancock, "Superpredator: The Media Myth That Demonized a Generation of Black Youth," The Marshall Project, November 20, 2020, themarshallproject.org/2020/11/20/superpredator-the-media-myth-that-demonized-a-generation-of-black-youth.

14. Laura I. Appleman, "Deviancy, Dependency, and Disability: The Forgotten History of Eugenics and Mass Incarceration," *Duke Law Journal* 68, no. 3 (2018): 62; Barry Godfrey and Steven Soper, "Prison records from 1800s Georgia show mass incarceration's racially charged beginnings," The Conversation, May 22, 2018, theconversation.com/prison-records-from-1800s-georgia-show-mass-incarcerations-racially-charged-beginnings-96612.

15. J. Money et al., "47,XYY and 46,XY Males with Antisocial and/or Sex-Offending Behavior: Antiandrogen Therapy plus Counseling," *Psychoneuroendocrinology* 1, no. 2 (1975): 165–78.

16. Claus Wiedeking et al., "Follow-up of 11 XYY Males with Impulsive and/or Sex-Offending Behaviour," *Psychological Medicine* 9, no. 2 (1979): 287–92.

17. Robert D. Miller, "Forced Administration of Sex-Drive Reducing Medications to Sex Offenders: Treatment or Punishment," *Psychology, Public Policy, and Law, Sex Offenders: Scientific, Legal, and Policy Perspectives* 4, no. 1–2 (1998): 175–99; Daniel B. Wood, "States Are Rushing to Curb Sex Crimes," *Christian Science Monitor* (1996): 4; David Boyers, "Review of Selected 1996 California Legislation," *Pacific Law Journal* 28 (1997): 740; Edward A. Fitzgerald, "Chemical Castration: MPA Treatment of the Sexual Offender," *American Journal of Criminal Law* 18, nos. 1–6 (1990); and Jason O. Runckel, "Abuse It and Lose It: A Look at California's Mandatory Chemical Castration Law," *Pacific Legal Journal* 28 (1997): 547.

18. John F. Stinneford, "Incapacitation Through Maiming: Chemical Castration, the Eighth Amendment, and the Denial of Human Dignity," *University of St. Thomas Law Journal* 3 (2006): 559–99.

19. Vincent J. Schodolski, "California Passes Chemical Castration Law," *The Washington Post*, August 31, 1996; Linda Beckman, "Chemical Castration: Constitutional Issues of Due Process, Equal Protection, and Cruel and Unusual Punishment," *West Virginia Law Review* 100, no. 4 (1998); and "Constitutional Law. Due Process and Equal Protection. California Becomes First State to Require Chemical Castration of Certain Sex Offenders. Act of September 17, 1996, Ch. 596, 1996 Cal. Stat. 92 (To Be Codified at Cal. Penal Code § 645)," *Harvard Law Review* 110, no. 3 (1997): 799–804.

20. Max Vanzi, "Assembly OKs Castration Drug for Molesters," *Los Angeles Times*, August 31, 1996.

21. Raymond M. Wood et al., "Psychological assessment, treatment, and outcome with sex offenders," *Behavioral Sciences & the Law* 18, no. 1 (2000): 23–41.

22. Madeline Carter and Leilah Gilligan, "Center for Sex Offender Management (CSOM)," The Center for Effective Public Policy, 2022, cepp.com/project/center-for-sex-offender-management-csom.

23. Matthew V. Daley, "A Flawed Solution to the Sex Offender Situation in the United States: The Legality of Chemical Castration for Sex Offenders," *Indiana Health Law Review* 5, no. 1 (2008): 88.

24. Corey G. Johnson, "Female Inmates Sterilized in California Prisons without Approval," *Reveal*, July 7, 2013, revealnews.org/article/female-inmates-sterilized-in-california-prisons-without-approval.

25. Ibid.

26. Ibid.

27. Hunter Schwarz, "Following Reports of Forced Sterilization of Female Prison Inmates, California Passes Ban," *The Washington Post*, September 26, 2014.

28. Colin Dwyer, "Judge Promises Reduced Jail Time If Tennessee Inmates Get Vasectomies," NPR, The Two-Way, July 21, 2017, npr.org/sections/thetwo-way/2017/07/21/538598008/judge-promises-reduced-jail-time-if-tennessee-inmates-get-vasectomies.

29. Elise B. Adams, "Voluntary Sterilization of Inmates for Reduced Prison Sentences," *Duke Journal of Gender Law & Policy* 26, no. 23 (2018): 23–44.

30. Tom Jackman, "Judge Suggests Drug-Addicted Woman Get Sterilized before Sentencing, and She Does," *The Washington Post*, February 8, 2018.

31. Sheila Burke, "Nashville Prosecutors Require Sterilization as Part of Plea Deals," Associated Press, in *The Boston Globe*, March 29, 2015.

32. Haley Smith, "Common Enemy and Political Opportunity Leave Archaically Modern Sentencing Unchecked: The Unconstitutionality of Louisiana's Chemical Castration Statute," *Loyola Law Review* 59 (2013): 211–66.

33. "Louisiana Has Highest Incarceration Rate in the World; ACLU Seeks Changes," American Civil Liberties Union, December 11, 2008, aclu.org/press-releases/louisiana-has-highest-incarceration-rate-world-aclu-seeks-changes.

34. Elizabeth Thomas, "Alabama Governor Signs Chemical Castration for Child Sex Offenders Bill," ABC11 Raleigh-Durham, June 11, 2019, abc11.com/alabama-governor-signs-chemical-castration-for-child-sex-offenders-bill-/5341620.

35. *State of Louisiana v. Lance S. Barton*, 319 So.3d 907 (Court of Appeal of Louisiana, Third Circuit, May 5, 2021).

36. Nick Reynolds, "Republican Looks to Lessen Prison Time for Drug Users Who Get Sterilized," *Newsweek*, December 7, 2022.

21. Newgenics?

1. Lee Rainie et al., "AI and Human Enhancement: Americans' Openness Is Tempered by a Range of Concerns," Pew Research Center: Internet, Science & Tech, March 17, 2022, pewresearch.org/internet/2022/03/17/ai-and-human-enhancement-americans-openness-is-tempered-by-a-range-of-concerns.

2. Paul Lombardo, "The 'Negro Children' at Tuskegee: The Banality of Eugenics," *Undark*, April 4, 2016, undark.org/2016/04/04/the-banality-of-eugenics-tuskegee.

3. Jerry Lambe, "'Like an Experimental Concentration Camp': Whistleblower Complaint Alleges Mass Hysterectomies at ICE Detention Center," *Law & Crime*, September 14, 2020, lawandcrime.com/high-profile/like-an-experimental-concentration-camp-whistleblower-complaint-alleges-mass-hysterectomies-at-ice-detention-center/; Jose Olivares and John Washington, "'A Silent Pandemic': Nurse at ICE Facility Blows the Whistle on Coronavirus Dangers," *The Intercept*, September 14, 2020, theintercept.com/2020/09/14/ice-detention-center-nurse-whistleblower.

4. "Coronavirus in Georgia | Latest Data for Sept. 20, 2020," 11Alive, September 20, 2020, 11alive.com/article/news/health/coronavirus/coronavirus-numbers/coronavirus-numbers-georgia-sept-20-2020/85-e76686ab-4895-4396-9381-bc1105448f31.

5. Meagan Platt, "Press Release: Whistleblowing Nurse from Detention Center in Georgia Reports Unsafe Practices That Promote the Spread of COVID-19 in ICE Detention," Government Accountability Project, September 14, 2020, whistleblower.org/press-release/press-release-whistleblowing-nurse-from-detention-center-in-georgia-reports-unsafe-practices-that-promote-the-spread-of-covid-19-in-ice-detention.

6. Jose Olivares and John Washington, "'A Silent Pandemic,'" op. cit.

7. Project South, Georgia Detention Watch, Georgia Latino Alliance for Human Rights, and South Georgia Immigrant Support Network, "Re: Lack of Medical Care, Unsafe Work Practices, and Absence of Adequate Protection Against COVID-19 for Detained Immigrants and Employees Alike at the Irwin County Detention Center," September 14, 2020, projectsouth.org/wp-content/uploads/2020/09/OIG-ICDC-Complaint-1.pdf.

8. Priyanka Bhatt et al., "Violence & Violation: Medical Abuse of Immigrants Detained at the Irwin County Detention Center," Harvard Immigration and Refugee Clinic and HLS Immigration Project, September 2021, harvardimmigrationclinic.org/files/2021/09/IrwinReport_FINAL.pdf.

9. Tina Vásquez, "ICE Is Now Detaining Women at One of the Nation's Most Deadly Facilities," Prism, February 2, 2021, prismreports.org/2021/02/02/ice-now-detaining-women-at-one-of-nations-most-deadly-facilities.

10. Ana Popovich, "DHS OIG Releases Report on Conduct at Irwin County Detention Center, Target of Whistleblower Complaints in 2020," Whistleblower Network News, January 13, 2022, whistleblowersblog.org/government-whistleblowers/dhs-oig-releases-report-on-conduct-at-irwin-county-detention-center-target-of-whistleblower-complaints-in-2020.

11. The Facility (2021), written and directed by Seth Freed Wessler, fieldofvision.org/the-facility.

12. Rebecca M. Kluchin, "Fit to Be Tied? Sterilization and Reproductive Rights in America, 1960–1984," PhD dissertation, Carnegie Mellon University (2004).

13. Greg Sargent, "Behind Tucker Carlson and J.D. Vance, a Revolt against the GOP Unfolds," The Washington Post, March 22, 2022.

Image Credits

All images are public domain, unless otherwise noted.

Page 9: Wellcome Library, London. Copyrighted work available under CC BY 4.0.

Pages 18, 70 (right), and 107: Photograph by the author.

Page 19: Courtesy of the Oneida Community Mansion House, catalog/accession no. A157. Thank you to Tom Guiler.

Page 26: Creative Commons Attribution-Share Alike 4.0 International license.

Page 33: Getty Images/ilbusca, DigitalVision Vectors.

Page 35: Courtesy of the Internet Archive.

Page 49: Ian Alexander, CC BY-SA 4.0.

Page 62: Courtesy of the Law Unit of Connecticut State Library and Museum of Connecticut History.

Page 69: Courtesy of Mary Washington College, Department of History and American Studies.

Pages 72, 78, 80, and 84: Created by Beth Bugler, based on information provided by the author and Benjamin Williams.

Page 76: The Harry H. Laughlin Papers, papers E-1-3, Truman State University.

Page 85: The *Los Angeles Times* Photographic Collection at the UCLA Library. CC BY 4.0.

Page 89: Courtesy of the *Santa Cruz Sentinel*.

Page 103: Arthur Estabrook Papers, Special Collections & Archives, University at Albany, SUNY.

Page 114: Courtesy of the Galton Papers, UCL Library Services, Special Collections.

Page 120: W. E. B. Du Bois Papers, Robert S. Cox Special Collections and University Archives Research Center, UMass Amherst Libraries.

Page 129: Courtesy of the University of Illinois at Urbana-Champaign Library, Urbana, IL, and the Library of Congress.

Page 131: The Harry H. Laughlin Papers, Truman State University, Lantern Slides, Brown Box, 1706.

Page 132: From Frank Gary Brooks, "Selling the Future Short," *Bios* 2, no. 3 (1931): 151–55. Recreated by Beth Bugler.

Page 139: Truman State University. Recreated by Beth Bugler.

Pages 143 and 172: Created by Beth Bugler, based on information provided by the author.

Pages 148, 151, 154, 226, and 237: Courtesy of the Library of Congress.

Page 160: Courtesy of Universitätsbibliothek Heidelberg, CC BY-SA 3.0 DE.

Page 163: Bundesarchiv, Bild 183-1998-0817-502/CC BY-SA 3.0

Page 174: Courtesy of Bundesarchiv.

Page 184: Keystone-France/Gamma-Keystone via Getty Images.

Page 189: Courtesy of Museum of Menstruation and Women's Health/ Harry Finley.

Page 194: Rockefeller Family records, photographs, series 1007, Rockefeller Archive Center. CC BY 4.0.

Page 197: Courtesy of Brigham and Women's Archives, Francis A. Countway Library, Harvard University.

Page 204: Courtesy of Princeton University Library Special Collections.

Page 209: Max Roser, CC BY-SA.

Page 216: This file is a copyrighted work of the Government of India, licensed under the Government Open Data License - India (GODL).

Page 217: From *The Limits to Growth* (1972), page 124, figure 35. CC BY-SA 4.0. Recreated by Beth Bugler.

Page 218: Courtesy of Clpro2. CC BY-SA 3.0.

Page 227: Courtesy of the Amistad Research Center.

Page 240: Courtesy of the American Indian Digital History Archive.

Page 245: Courtesy of *The Washington Post*.

Page 258: Anthony Crider, Creative Commons Attribution 2.0 Generic.

Acknowledgments

Every book takes a village. Here are the people in my book-village. Thank you for lending me your knowledge, wisdom, effort, and thoughtfulness.

Inspiration: Chris Hamlin encouraged me to write this book while we were sitting on his porch in 2010. I told him there were eugenics histories already, that everyone already knew this stuff, and, by the way, who was I to try to attempt a book on this? When, a decade later, Richard Dawkins tweeted a pro-eugenics howler just before COVID-19 shut down the world, I realized Chris was right—which, of course, he usually is.

Suppliers of images, facts, arguments, connections, and ideas: Jim Bindon, Subhadra Das, Harry Finley (Museum of Menstruation), Michael A. Flannery, Scott Gilbert, Thomas A. Guiler (Oneida), Beatrix Haußmann (Bundesarchiv), Lutz Kaelber, Lucy Kaufman, Matthew Lockwood, Stephanie McClure, Paul Wolff Mitchell, Jessica Murphy, Margaret Peacock, Josh Pederson, Juanjo Ponce Vázquez, Phillip R. Sloan, Jeremy Smith, Sonya Spillmann, Ellen Wayland-Smith, L. Jo Weaver, Benjamin Williams, Rob Wilson, and archivists at the US Holocaust Memorial Museum, the Cambridge University Library, the Weston Library at Oxford University, University College London, the British Library, the Library of Congress, National Archives in the US and UK, and the Eugenics Archive, Canada.

The patient and skilled team at The Experiment: Nick Cizek, Beth Bugler, Margie Guerra, Jennifer Hergenroeder, Ann Kirschner, Matthew Lore, Zachary Pace, Pamela Schechter, and Sophie Thompson.

Jane Dystel and the entire group at Dystel, Goderich & Bourret LLC.

Emotional support people/animals: Jimmy Mixon & The 603 Band; Bob, Shelley, Marianne, and fellow Alcovians; Andy, Brant, Brian, John, Brad, Barbara, Brooke, Greta, Will, Dewey, Frances Bacon, and Jinx.

Index

Copeland, Lammot du Pont, 199
crime: environmental causes of, 93–
    95; eugenics legislation to prevent,
    62–63; and habitual criminals,
    36, 68, 99, 228; and heredity,
    32–45, 60, 75, 246–53; and
    mental degeneration, 28; punitive
    sterilization for, 45, 62–63, 67–70,
    98–100, 228–30, 247–51; sex
    offenders, 98–99, 102–3, 250, 252;
    and Y-chromosome abnormalities,
    246–49. *See also* criminal
    anthropology; prisons
criminal anthropology, 32–45;
    brain dissections, 34–36; criminal
    insanity legal defense, 37–38;
    eugenics to solve degeneration,
    44–45; origins of, 32–34; and
    physical traits, 32–33, 39, 42–44;
    and racism, 40–42
The Criminal Man (Lombroso),
    40–41

Darrow, Clarence, 224
Darwin, Charles: and core narrative
    of eugenics, 131; and criminal
    anthropology, 33–34; and Galton's
    theories, 47, 53–54, 74; pangenesis
    theory of, 48–50, 53–54; and race,
    40; and selective breeding, 14, 17;
    on sexual selection, 55
Darwin, Leonard, 126–27, 136–37,
    158
Davenport, Charles B.: and Eugenics
    Records Office, 72–77; and
    German eugenics, 158–64, 169;
    and global eugenics network,
    126–27; at International Congress
    of Eugenics, New York, 130;
    and International Federation of
    Eugenics Organizations, 135;
    Japan, inspiration for eugenics in,
    144; and Permanent International
    Eugenics Commission, 158;
    at Race Betterment Society
    conference, 82–83
Davis v. Berry (1914), 99–101

degenerates. *See* white racial degeneration
Dégénérescence et criminalité ("Degeneracy
    and Criminality," Féré), 30
demographic changes, 8, 59, 218, 258. *See
    also* population control
Deng Xiaoping, 216
Department of Health, Education, and
    Welfare (HEW), 233–34, 241, 243
Depo-Provera (birth control), 232–34, 249,
    252, 255
*Descent of Man, and Selection in Relation to
    Sex* (Darwin), 40, 55
DiIulio, John J., Jr, 248
Disney, 208
Disraeli, Benjamin, 115
Djerassi, Carl, 189
Dobson, James C., 89
Dom Pedro II (emperor of Brazil), 141
Douglas, William O., 229–30
Doyle, Arthur Conan, 42–43
Draper, Wickliffe Preston, 166, 178,
    197–98
Draper, William H., Jr, 195, 199–200, 204
Draper Committee, 195–96
Dugdale, Richard L., 93–95, 129
Dulles, John Foster, 193–94
DuPont family, 199

East, Edward M., 226
Eastland, James O., 227
Economic Opportunity Act (1964), 231
Edgar, W. R., 62–64
Ehrenfels, Christian von, 113, 115–16
Ehrlich, Paul, 200, 203–10, 211
Eisenhower, Dwight D., 195–97, 199
Eisenstadt v. Baird (1972), 189–90
Emergency Quota Act (1921), 153
England, 46, 56, 57, 126, 160
*English Men of Science: Their Nature and
    Nurture* (Galton), 56
Entartung (Degeneration, Nordau), 63
environment: and brain shrinkage, 27;
    heredity vs., 29, 44–45, 93–95; race
    vs., 112; stress and behavior, 111; in
    Uruguay, interventions for, 148
environmental movement, 203, 205–6,
    210, 212

Paul IV (pope), 190
Pearl, Raymond, 225–26
Pearson, Karl, 57, 72–73
people with disabilities: euthanasia of, 171–73; German eugenics propaganda on, 167; and Greek and Roman infanticide, 16; and repeal of eugenics laws, 243; sterilization of, 233–34; as vulnerable population, 75
Permanent International Eugenics Commission, 158
Person, Karl, 57
Peru, 219–20
Philpott, Austin F., 99–100
Physical Deterioration Being Mainly an Indictment Against the Cities of the Time (Saleeby), 111
physical traits: and anthropometry, 129–30; and criminal anthropology, 32–33, 39, 42–44; and Cro-Magnon dominance, 129; head structure and mental degeneration, 28–29; International Congress of Eugenics exhibits on, 129–31; and Nazi eugenics movement, 163; and phrenology, 32, 34–35, 44; and scientific racism, 7
Pincus, Gregory, 187–90
Pinkerman-Uri, Connie Redbird, 241–42
Plato, 15–16, 74
Plecker, W. A., 141
Ploetz, Alfred, 158
Popenoe, Paul, 71, 83–86, 107
The Population Bomb (Ehrlich), 200, 203–10
The Population Bomb Is Everyone's Baby (Moore), 200
Population Connection, 204
population control, 181–220; in China, 216–19; and Draper Committee, 195–97; Wickliffe Drapper and financing of, 197–99; in India, 211–16; industrial complex of, 193–202; International Eugenics Congress on, 137; overpopulation leading to

revolutions, 193–95; in Peru, 219–20; and *The Population Bomb*, 203–10; and Population Council, 194–95; and Population Crisis Committee, 199–200, 204; through USAID and NGOs, 200–202; and World Population Congress, 164. *See also* Puerto Rico
Population Council, 194–95
Population Crisis Committee (PCC), 199–200, 204
population policy, 207–8
poverty, 231–45; children, birth control for, 232–35; communism and, 194–96, 200, 212; and environment, 93–95; forced sterilization for, 68; and heredity, 60, 90–91; and Indian Health Care Improvement Act, 237–42; legislation to counter, 231; polls on sterilization of poor women, 244–45; and repeal of eugenics laws, 242–44; sterilizations coerced during childbirth, 235–37, 239–41; and vulnerable populations, 75. *See also* burden of caring for unfit persons; population control
power dynamics, 5, 38–39, 44, 83
Priddy, Albert, 103–5
Principles of Human Heredity and Race Hygiene (Baur, Fischer, & Lenz), 163
prisons: chemical castrations in, 249–52; and criminal anthropology, 39; financial costs of, 60–61; heredity of crime in records of inmates, 36; imprisonment as eugenics, 249; medical trials in, 175; sterilizations in, 62, 67–70, 78–79, 98–101, 254–57; sterilizations to avoid, 227–28, 252–53
Problems of Human Reproduction (Popenoe), 87
The Progress of Eugenics (Saleeby), 112
propaganda on eugenics, 71, 158, 159, 161–63, 166–68
prostitution, 87
Public Citizen's Health Research Group (PCHRG), 238–39, 242
Public Health Services Act (1970), 231
Puerto Rico, 181–92; birth control promoted in, 182–83; labor strikes, 183–84; pharmaceutical testing in, 183, 187–90; population control in, 184–86;

velvet eugenics, 1–2, 254, 257
Verschuer, Otmar Freiherr, 177–78, 199
Vietnam, 200
Virginia, 70, 102–7, 243
viriculture (Galton), 55–58

Wagner, Richard, 112–13
War on Poverty, 231, 238
warrior gene, 248
Washington, 98–99
Washington v. Harper (1990), 249
Webb, James E., 195
Weinberger, Caspar, 234
welfare, 199, 228, 238
Wells, Charlotte Fowler, 34
Wells, H. G., 56, 58–59
Wessler, Seth Freed, 256–57
white racial degeneration, 22–32; and heredity, 27–30; perceived increase and fear of, 22–23; in popular novels, 30–31; race mixing as cause of, 23–27, 55, 112–13. *See also* family lineages
white supremacy: in core narrative of eugenics, 133–34, 138; and criminal anthropology, 40; and fears of weakness, 64, 116; and Galton's viriculture, 55–58; and nuclear family, 87–88; in post WWI Germany, 157–65; race mixing and, 23–27, 55, 112–13; race mixing to eliminate other races, 56, 140–42; and scientific racism, 7–8, 40, 116, 130, 226; and selective breeding, 81; and social Darwinism, 8; sterilization of degenerates to preserve, 106–7; in Switzerland, 147; and US immigration law, 150–54; and white replacement theory, 8, 258. *See also* population control; racial hierarchy and racism
Wilson, E. B., 226
Wilson, Woodrow, 153
Winship, Blanton, 183–84
Woman & Womanhood (Saleeby), 112

women: birth control and liberation of, 189–91, 200–202, 210; feminism and sexual revolution, 190–92, 210; involuntary sterilizations of, 186–87, 192, 199–200, 219, 227–29, 232–45, 250, 254–57; sexual preferences and hereditary traits, 40; women's rights movement, 19, 64
Wood, Alfred, 67
Woodhull, Victoria, 19–21, 74, 191
Wooten, Dawn, 254–55
World Bank, 201
World Conference on Women, Beijing (1995), 219
World Population Conference, Romania (1974), 209
World Population Congress of IUSIPP, Berlin (1935), 164
World War I, 130, 159, 162
World War II, 145. *See also* Holocaust; Nazi Germany
Wright, Albert O., 60–61

Yamanouchi Shigeo, 144
Y-chromosome abnormalities, 246–49

Zero Population Growth (ZPG) movement, 204, 208–9
Zola, Émile, 30–31
Zyklon-B, 173

About the Author

ERIK L. PETERSON, PhD, is associate provost and associate professor of the history of science and medicine at the University of Alabama. He publishes and teaches about the historical relationship between race and science in the US and abroad.

Also available in the Shortest History series

Trade Paperback Originals • $16.95 US | $21.95 CAN

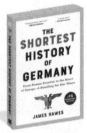
978-1-61519-569-5

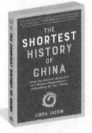
978-1-61519-820-7

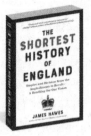
978-1-61519-814-6

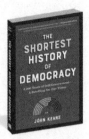
978-1-61519-896-2

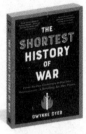
978-1-61519-930-3

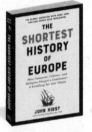
978-1-61519-914-3

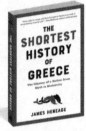
978-1-61519-948-8

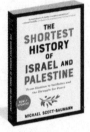
978-1-61519-950-1

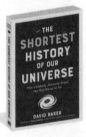
978-1-61519-973-0

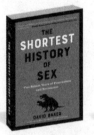
978-1-891011-34-4

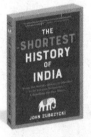
978-1-61519-997-6

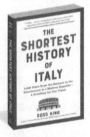
978-1-891011-45-0

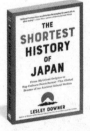
978-1-891011-66-5

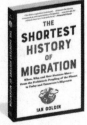
979-8-89303-060-0

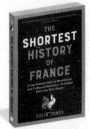
979-8-89303-012-9